A COMPREHENSIVE GUIDE TO

BREAST
AUGMENTATION

THE BEVERLY HILLS PLASTIC SURGERY SERIES

A COMPREHENSIVE GUIDE TO

BREAST
AUGMENTATION

DR. JOHN DIAZ

Board-Certified Plastic Surgeon

BEVERLY HILLS, CA

ISBN-13: 978-0-692-77032-0

Library of Congress Control Number: 2016916573

PRINTED IN THE USA

10 9 8 7 6 5 4 3 2 1

I dedicate this book to all patients
seeking breast augmentation.

TABLE OF CONTENTS

ACKNOWLEDGEMENTS

This book was inspired by my patients. It is often said that you learn as much from those you help as they learn from you. This could not be more true. Over the past decade, I have had the privilege of treating thousands of patients and have felt honored in helping them achieve the look they dreamed of. I especially enjoy having consultations with patients because I am able to connect on a personal level with people from all over the world and from all kinds of backgrounds. Most of all, the questions they pose and the requests they make drive me to constantly improve and refine my techniques to achieve excellence. For this, I am truly grateful.

I would like to thank my office staff—an incredible team of professionals who elevate my practice every day. Thanks to their help, I am able to deliver superior care and results to my patients.

Also, I would like to thank Lawrence Ineno. He is a superb editor. For the past two years, Lawrence has guided me in taking this book from an idea to a reality. His insights, comments, and suggestions were invaluable. Without him, this book would not be the same.

I would like to thank my family. My parents taught me by example the value of hard work, dedication, and sacrifice. My brother, sister, nieces, and nephews daily remind me of the importance of family and making every day count. I push myself every day to make them proud.

Lastly, I would like to thank my incredible wife, Ursula. She has been unbelievably supportive and encouraging throughout the entire writing process. This book was made better because of her feedback and suggestions. Our marriage is the rock and foundation of my life. Her love gives me the strength to believe in myself and encourages me every single day to be the best man that I can be.

INTRODUCTION

Emily arrived at my office for her initial breast augmentation appointment. When I entered the consultation room to meet her, she sat firmly planted in her chair, hands tightly clasped together on her lap, and sweat beading on her forehead.

As with every meeting, I introduced myself and then learned more about her: What result did she seek, was there any particular implant she wanted to know more about, and what was her surgery timeframe? A combination of nervousness and uncertainty caused her to stammer through her responses.

At one point, as I was asking her a question, she interrupted me. "Dr. Diaz, I'm scared. I mean I've done tons of Internet research, but it's left me feeling confused and totally overwhelmed," Emily said. Like many women seeking breast augmentation, she was anxious about the entire process.

Although the Internet has provided consumers more information than ever about plastic surgery procedures, I've found many online resources that are confusing, misleading, or downright inaccurate. You can certainly find great plastic surgery sites, but there are also many terrible ones.

Contradictory content (one so-called expert says one thing, while another says something else), questionable sources (non-experts share their personal stories and charlatans masquerade as plastic surgery experts), and resources with inherent conflicts of interest make it tough—if not downright impossible—to know where to access reliable and accurate information. In fact, Emily's confession is one I've heard countless times throughout my plastic surgery career.

The vast majority of patients I meet with (in fact, I'd estimate over 90 percent) are misguided or misinformed or both about breast augmentation. My goal is always to shed light on areas that confuse patients and address their biggest concerns.

Unfortunately, as a solo practitioner based in Beverly Hills, I can only help a limited number of patients. That is what inspired me to write The Beverly Hills Plastic Surgery Series. These pages are an essential resource for millions of women across the country who, every day, spend innumerable hours online, speak to friends and family, and consult with physicians about breast augmentation.

In this book, you'll receive the most up-to-date, accurate, and patient-friendly information about breast augmentation—from the preparation you need to perform before even scheduling a consultation to tips to experiencing the best result possible. I'll answer inquiries such as "How do I find the best doctor for me?" "What are my implant options and what are each one's strengths and weaknesses?" and "How much will this cost?" I'll also dispel common myths and misconceptions.

This book follows the patients-first client service model I've developed. It makes certain that I answer every possible question a patient has and prevents misunderstandings. I've found that structuring my service model this way ensures that all my patients receive consistent, high-quality service and their goals are met.

I love my work, and I'm passionate about improving my patients' lives. And my patients appreciate how I invest time addressing their concerns and explain complicated surgical procedures in a straight-forward and easy-to-understand way. My goal is to provide you a similar degree of integrity, clarity, and expertise.

In the past, you may have worked with a fitness trainer, therapist, or both to support you and address your biggest concerns. Similarly, think of this book as having a Beverly Hills plastic surgeon by your side guiding you through every step of your breast augmentation. So let's get started!

CHAPTER 1

BEFORE THE CONSULTATION

In this chapter, you'll learn:

- what a breast augmentation is;
- whether you're a good candidate for breast augmentation;
- essential subjective and objective questions to ask yourself before a consultation.

Real Conversations

"Sarah, you need to stop thinking about this and call right now!" Brittany told her best friend. For nearly a year, Sarah had considered undergoing breast augmentation. At Brittany's insistence, Sarah finally decided to phone my office. She spoke with my administrative assistant and asked to schedule a consultation.

"We'd love to have you come to our office. Dr. Diaz's next available appointment is in three weeks," she said.

"Three weeks? Can't we meet tomorrow?" Sarah asked.

Preparation Is Key: Don't Rush

From fast food ("Your pizza delivered in thirty minutes or less!") to fast diets ("Lose twenty pounds in two weeks!"), we've grown accustomed to getting what we want *right now!*

But when it comes to breast augmentation, you should never rush your decision. In Sarah's case, prior to meeting with any plastic surgeon, she needed to do her homework. This is because the consultation is a very important step in the breast augmentation process. It's your opportunity to learn as much as possible about your prospective surgeon, your numerous implant options, and the procedure itself. The better prepared for the consultation, the more you'll benefit from it.

Thus, rather than view the consultation as the first step in Sarah's discovery process, she needed to conduct more research on her own. At the same time, with so much information available to her, deciding where to begin would be a daunting task. In this chapter, you'll learn the essential information you'll need to conduct your search.

What Is Breast Augmentation?

Simply put, breast augmentation is the enhancement of the breast's volume. Breast implants come in a variety of shapes and sizes. Each provides slightly different results, but the bottom line is breast augmentation primarily increases your breast size.

Breast augmentation can't change preexisting asymmetries in the breast shape or nipple position. This will be covered in chapter 9.

Is Breast Augmentation for Me?

The best candidates are women who have given their surgery decision careful thought. Over my career performing thousands of procedures, I've identified key aspects patients focus on that have yielded the most satisfying results. They are as follows:

- **Self-Improvement**—They seek to undergo breast augmentation for themselves, rather than for someone else.

- **Thorough Research**—They carefully consider their decision and objectively assess the pros and cons of their surgical options.

- **Realistic Expectations**—They understand and accept the limitations of their procedure. For example, they realize the existing shape of their breast will influence and perhaps limit their result.

Be Honest with Yourself: Five Self-Assessment Questions

"What kind of look would you like to have?" I asked Sarah during her consultation.

"Natural . . . I definitely don't want anyone to notice I've had my breasts done," she said.

As a result, Sarah expressed a C-cup would probably meet her needs.

"Great, do you have any photos to show me?" I asked.

I often encourage patients to bring pictures of friends or magazine images reflecting their breast augmentation preferences.

Sarah pulled her iPad from her purse. On her Instagram account were models with *Bay Watch*-size breasts. At that moment, I knew what she *said she wanted* failed to align with the result she *really wanted.*

While a skilled plastic surgeon will help you determine the outcome you seek by asking questions, describing your options, and taking accurate measurements, you must express your wants clearly. Identifying them ahead of time is essential to having a successful consultation. After all, a surgeon can only help you achieve your goals if you have determined them yourself.

In order to identify your goals, ask yourself the following questions:

1.   Why am I seeking breast augmentation?

2.   Is this a good time for me to have surgery?

3.   How much larger do I want my breasts to be?

4.   What are my short-term and long-term goals?

5.   What look do I want to achieve?

WHY AM I SEEKING BREAST AUGMENTATION?

Make sure your motivation to undergo a breast augmentation comes from within. In other words, never undergo any cosmetic surgery procedure because someone, other than you, is pressuring you to do so. In my experience, I've found you most likely won't be satisfied with the outcome if you are seeking it primarily because someone else wants it for you. This is because the result reflects another person's aesthetic preference and not necessarily yours.

IS THIS A GOOD TIME FOR ME TO HAVE SURGERY?

Undergoing breast augmentation can be one of the most exciting and life-enhancing decisions you'll ever make. With that said, you should always keep in mind a breast augmentation is a true medical procedure and a major decision. As with any major decision, maintaining objectivity is key to experiencing a satisfying result. Your best decision-making ability comes when you're calm, able to think clearly, and not driven solely by emotions.

That's why I recommend avoiding breast augmentation during significant life changes. Examples include romantic breakups, divorce, and any emotional loss that could influence your objectivity. If any of these scenarios describe your current state, consider waiting until your life circumstances feel steady and firmly within your control.

HOW MUCH LARGER DO I WANT MY BREASTS TO BE?

Determining your goals will help you make decisions that provide the immediate and long-term results you seek. Thus, you should invest time thinking through your options. For example do you want a B, C, or D cup?

If you're not sure, go online and view images of models or celebrities that have the breast size you would like. (See figures 1.1 and 1.2.) Once you find photos reflecting the size that appeals to you, save them on your mobile device or print them. These can be useful guides during your consultation.

Another common approach is to ask your friends for help. Speak with people you know who have undergone breast augmentation or know someone who has. They may be able to offer advice and feedback about implant sizes and surgeons.

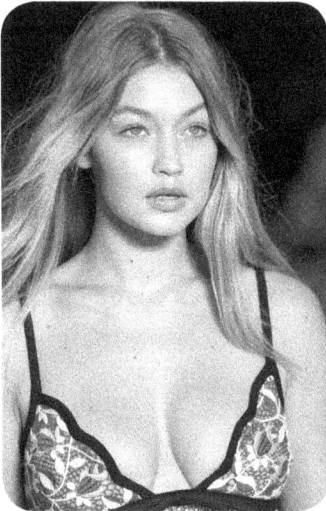

FIGURE 1.1 Gigi Hadid. Estimated to have C cup breasts. (Gigi Hadid is not a patient, and I have never treated her.)

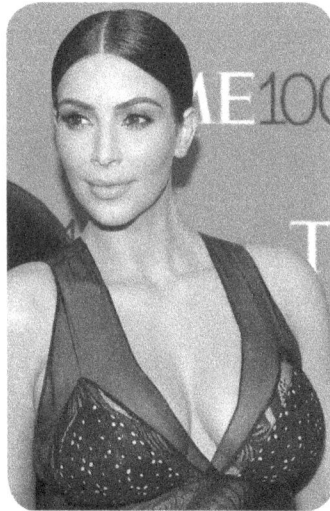

FIGURE 1.2 Kim Kardashian. Estimated to have full D cup breasts. (Kim Kardashian is not a patient, and I have never treated her.)

By having a general idea of your target cup size, your consultation will be more productive.

WHAT ARE MY SHORT-TERM AND LONG-TERM GOALS?

When it comes to goal setting, always make sure you consider how the cup size you seek will look in one, five, ten, and twenty years. While double-D breasts may look amazing on your college-age body, they may be less appealing later in life or after you've had children.

WHAT LOOK DO I WANT TO ACHIEVE?

Examples include an augmented and round look or a more natural look. Review photos of friends and celebrities with breasts that reflect the result you seek.

Keep in mind the bra type the person is wearing will affect the appearance of her breasts. For example, a push-up bra will make the breasts appear larger and rounder than they actually are. Also, the way a woman holds her arms will influence how her breasts look—lingerie and swimsuit models regularly position their arms close to their chest because doing so pushes their breasts together, which creates more cleavage. (See figure 1.3.)

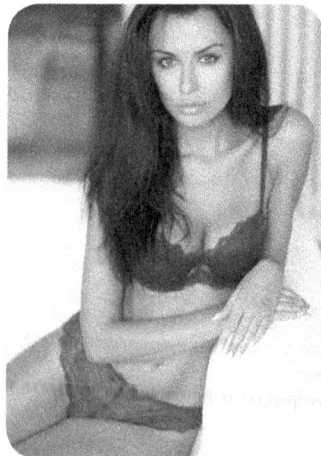

FIGURE 1.3 Lingerie tends to push breasts together and higher. This, in combination with the woman's pose and the position of her arms, accentuates her cleavage. (This is a model and not a patient.)

In general, natural breasts don't have cleavage unless they're pushed or pressed together with a bra, outer clothing, or both. Also, the larger and rounder the breasts you seek are, the less natural they will look.

In chapter 5, we'll explore the answer to this question in greater depth.

Plastic Surgery Nuts and Bolts: Five Practical Questions

The following address objective considerations you must make. They are just as important as subjective self-assessment questions you just learned:

1. When should I schedule a consultation?

2. Where will I have my procedure performed?

3. How do I budget for breast augmentation?

4. Who should be my surgeon?

5. Who will help me during the recovery?

WHEN SHOULD I SCHEDULE A CONSULTATION?

Ideally, your consultation should take place a few weeks before you plan to undergo breast augmentation. If your consultation takes place a year or more or even only five or six months *before* you commit, you're wasting your time. This is because by the time you're ready to schedule your procedure, your preferences or life circumstances may have changed for numerous reasons, which means you'll have to start the preparation process over again. Why is this?

Planning for a breast augmentation requires detailed research and keeping track of a significant amount of information. By the time

MON	TUE	WED	THU	FRI	SAT	SUN
28	29	30	1	2	3	4
5	6	7	8	9	10	11
12	13	14	15	16	17	18
19	20	21	22	23	24	25
26	27	28	29	30	31	

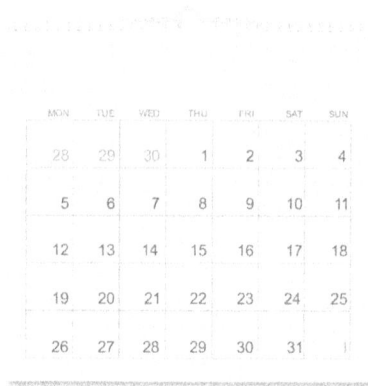

months have passed, you'll have forgotten what you researched and discussed during the initial consultation. For instance, I've met with patients who had preliminary consultations and then met with me six months or more later. They were now finally ready to book their surgery. The following is how a conversation such as this would go:

"In my notes, I see you wanted moderate-plus profile implants when we met six months ago," I say.

"I did?" the patient asks. "I don't remember why I said that. Can you review that for me again?"

The patient's confusion means she has to begin the process of assessing the pros and cons of each implant—just as she did months ago.

WHERE WILL I HAVE MY PROCEDURE PERFORMED?

You may have heard of medical tourism. This describes patients who undergo procedures far from their homes. I have patients who travel from all over the country and world to have their breast augmentations performed in my Beverly Hills surgery center. (See figure 1.4.)

If you're planning to travel in order to have your breast augmentation, you should consult with your surgeon and his or her staff.

They should provide you a checklist that includes travel arrangements and pre-op and post-op considerations you'll need to make.

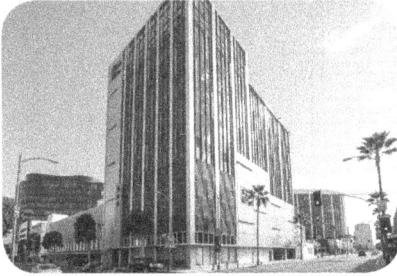

FIGURE 1.4 The Beverly Hills office building where Dr. John Diaz's practice is located.

HOW DO I BUDGET FOR BREAST AUGMENTATION?

Breast augmentation is a cosmetic elective procedure, which means it is *not* covered by health insurance. As a result, you must take care of all costs. The dollar amount of a breast augmentation depends on the surgeon's experience, reputation, and geographic location. In regards to geography, maintaining a surgical practice in sought-after and densely populated areas such as Beverly Hills, Manhattan, and San Francisco is more expensive than in other parts of the United States. Costs range from $3,500 to $12,000.

Once you've figured out the cost, you'll need to determine how you'll pay for your breast augmentation. Options include cash, a credit card, a loan, a cosmetic surgery gift card—yes, these exist—and any combination of these. If you take a loan out for your surgery, you can use cosmetic surgery credit cards, regular credit cards, and bank loans.

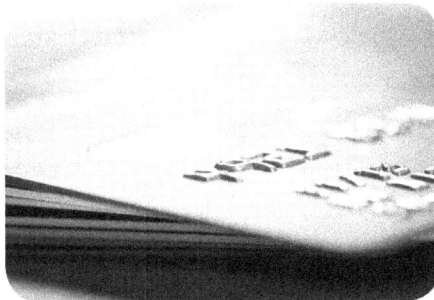

In order to benefit the most from your initial consultation, make sure you have identified how you'll pay for your surgery. For instance, if you're planning to finance your breast augmentation, knowing your credit score will save you time.

A low score will deem you ineligible to obtain a line of credit for your procedure. In this scenario, you would be better served postponing your consultation until you have met the credit score thresholds. If your credit score is high and you qualify for a line of credit, evaluate loan interest rates and carefully review rules and restrictions.

WHO SHOULD BE MY SURGEON?

This is the highest priority question of all. While the previous questions are critical, your surgeon's skill is the single most important factor to ensure a safe and successful result. Selecting your doctor is so important that the next chapter's sole focus is how to find the right surgeon.

WHO WILL HELP ME DURING THE RECOVERY?

If you're having your breast augmentation performed close to home, you should coordinate the surgery to fit the schedule of friends, family, and anyone else who will help in your recovery. You'll definitely count on their support, so plan accordingly.

Whether you're traveling or staying local, be sure to think ahead. Make sure you have arranged to take time off from work or school to recover. Your surgeon will provide specific recovery timelines based on your particular circumstances. In general, you'll need about a week off from work or school. You'll more about this in chapter 11.

Summary

- Breast augmentation is an enhancement of the breast's volume. The procedure will make your breasts larger, but it won't significantly change the shape or correct major asymmetries.

- The best candidates for breast augmentation are those who focus on self-improvement, thorough research, and realistic expectations.

- Being honest with yourself and clearly identifying your goals from the start is key to preparing for a successful consultation.

- Before scheduling your consultation, you should consider when and where you plan to have your procedure performed, determine your budget, have a clear plan to assess the quality of your prospective surgeon, and identify who will help you during your recovery.

Now that you've learned what you need to address before ever scheduling a breast augmentation consultation, in the next chapter, I'll guide you through your search. With literally thousands of options, finding a doctor with superior skill and patient service is overwhelming and confusing. From your initial Internet search to your first face-to-face appointment, I'll provide specific tools to help you identify the surgeon who will best meet your particular needs.

Breast Augmentation Myth

> The surgeon will tell me everything I need to know during the consultation. I don't really have to give this much thought.

Although it is true that excellent and caring surgeons, like myself, will provide you with all the information you need, you will have a much more productive and positive experience if you prepare ahead of time. Asking yourself the questions in this chapter *before* you come in for a consultation will help clarify your needs and goals.

There is a lot of information you will cover during the consultation, and many decisions you will need to make during your appointment. Knowing the information and having a good idea about what you would like your result to look like will make this process much easier and more pleasant.

CHAPTER 2

FINDING THE RIGHT SURGEON

In this chapter, you'll learn:

- what board certification in plastic surgery means and why it is important;

- information to look for when researching a surgeon;

- what to look for when reviewing websites and review sites on surgeons.

Real Conversations

By the time Amanda booked an introductory consultation to see me, she had already met two other surgeons. She was eager to select her final doctor and move forward with her procedure.

"One of the surgeons I visited recommended I go as big as possible," she said.

"But is that what *you* want? After all, my recommendations are always based on the result *you* are looking for, not what anyone else thinks," I said.

"Dr. Diaz, in all honesty, I didn't want to be that big. But he was pressuring me, and I thought I should follow his advice. After all, he's the expert," Amanda said.

"Can you tell me who the surgeon was?" I asked.

Amanda provided me his name. I then performed a Google search. Together, we scrolled through his website. I looked carefully for his resume, which wasn't readily accessible. Despite it being buried deeply within his site, I was able to find it.

"Did you know he wasn't a plastic surgeon?" I asked.

"Really? But I distinctly remember him telling me he was board certified," she said.

The doctor didn't lie. According to his website he was board certified—albeit not in plastic surgery. I then input his name on the American Board of Medical Specialties website. The site verified he was, in fact, board certified . . . but in ear, nose, and throat (ENT) surgery.

"That news is really disappointing. With so much information out there about breast augmentation, it's really difficult to know what to look for and whom to believe," she said.

Information Overload

The Internet has given women seeking breast augmentation unprecedented amounts of content to research. But the blessing of abundant data can also be a curse: How do you separate valuable information from its superfluous and sometimes even harmful counterpart? With millions of breast augmentation websites, where do you begin your search?

In this chapter, you'll learn straightforward strategies to evaluate a surgeon's qualification, reputation, and skill *before* you ever schedule an appointment. Done right, the Internet is an efficient and effective tool to guide you in your preliminary search.

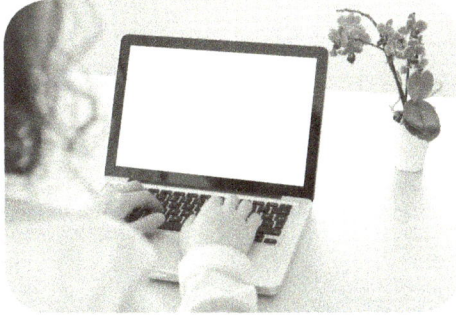

What Is Board Certification?

Think of board certification as a screening process that confirms a doctor is a safe and competent physician. The medical field has many different board certifications. The American Board of Medical Specialties (ABMS) identifies and oversees twenty-four of them. For example, a physician can be board certified in plastic surgery, otolaryngology (often called ENT), gynecology, family medicine, emergency medicine, or dermatology, to name a few.

Once a doctor is board certified, he or she is board certified across the country. A doctor can also have more than one board certification if he or she has completed more than one training program. You'll often hear this described as "double board certified" or even "triple board certified."

From a legal perspective, board certification isn't required to practice medicine. In fact, you'd probably be surprised to learn that many household names in plastic surgery and so-called celebrity surgeons are *not* board certified in anything, let alone plastic surgery. After reading this chapter, you'll easily be able to perform your own research and determine if the doctor is board certified or not.

Board Certification in Plastic Surgery

The training to become a board-certified plastic surgeon is as lengthy and rigorous as the training required to become a brain or heart surgeon. And statistics show that being accepted to a plastic surgery training program is *more difficult and competitive* than brain surgery and heart surgery programs.

Based on the experience I have meeting hundreds of patients every year in my office, I bet this information comes as a surprise. But it's true.

If popular media depictions of medical procedures appeared on a continuum, on one end you would have brain surgery, which is typically portrayed as heroic and a matter of life and death. And on the other end you would have plastic surgery, which often appears as frivolous and fun.

Unfortunately, the proliferation of doctors who blur the line between plastic surgeon and media personality, as well as reality and non-reality medical TV shows, has over-simplified the rigors and complexities of plastic surgery medical training—largely for the sake of creating a description packaged for mass consumption and entertainment.

Indeed, one of the downsides to plastic surgery's celebrity status is the downplay of the work required to become a board-certified plastic surgeon. The following description aims to set the record straight.

In order to become a board-certified plastic surgeon, a person must have done the following:

- Completed four years of college

- Scored highly on an extremely difficult Medical College Admissions Test (MCAT)

- Graduated from a four-year medical school

- Passed two challenging United States Medical Licensing Exams (USMLE)

- Applied and been accepted into a general surgical training program

- Completed three to five years of general surgery training (also called residency)

- Scored highly on the General Surgery In-Service Exam during residency

- Applied and been accepted into a plastic surgery training program

- Finished three years of plastic surgery training

- Scored highly on the Plastic Surgery In-Service Exam

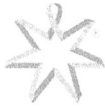

American Board of Plastic Surgery
ABMS Maintenance of Certification®
Certification Matters

And this list represents only the beginning. In addition, many surgeons complete one or more years of training in a plastic surgery subspecialty. This includes cosmetic surgery, craniofacial surgery, microsurgery, burn surgery, and hand surgery.

Once a doctor has met all the necessary requirements, he or she must take two final exams that take two to three years in total to complete. These are the written and oral exams. The written test evaluates a doctor's overall knowledge of plastic surgery. The oral exam comprises an evaluation of the surgeon's work by plastic surgery experts. Applicants must submit a year's worth of their patient and surgery experience. They are judged on their skill and their patient care and outcomes.

Only those who pass this final two-part stage of grueling exams earn the honor of calling themselves board-certified plastic surgeons. In other words, board-certified plastic surgeons undergo from eleven to sixteen years of medical training *after* they've earned their four-year college degree.

Not All Board Certifications Are Alike

Unfortunately, making sure your prospective surgeon has the proper credentials to perform breast augmentation is confusing. Just as Amanda discovered at the start of this chapter, your prospective surgeon should be not only generally board certified but also board certified specifically in *plastic surgery.*

You'll hear doctors who perform breast augmentations use many titles. Some call themselves plastic surgeons. Others use cosmetic surgeon. And you may also hear aesthetic plastic surgeon. Unfortunately, because so many doctors are taking advantage of the public's confusion over plastic surgeon designations, doctors regularly misuse these designations.

Specifically, anyone can call himself or herself a cosmetic surgeon. Thus the term *board-certified cosmetic surgeon* is particularly problematic.

Among the ABMS's twenty-four board certifications the organization oversees, which you learned about earlier, *there's no such thing as board certification in cosmetic surgery.* So when a doctor says, "I'm a board-certified cosmetic surgeon," I believe the doctor is actively duping the public or, in the least, is taking advantage of and fueling public misconception.

In other words, a doctor can get away with calling himself or herself a board certified cosmetic surgeon because what the doctor most often really is saying is, "I'm board certified in something. I'm just not stating what it is. And I'm conveniently adding 'cosmetic surgery' to the end of my made-up title." His or her unmentioned board certification could be any of the twenty-three other certifications. Many doctors use this loophole to trick prospective patients.

On the other hand, only surgeons who are board certified in plastic surgery can identify themselves as *a board-certified plastic surgeon*. If a doctor is caught calling himself or herself a board-certified plastic surgeon when this isn't the case, he or she is subject to swift and harsh disciplinary action by a state medical board. And that goes for all false claims of any board certification.

You'd hope these strict usage guidelines would keep surgeons from making fraudulent claims about their credentials. Unfortunately, some surgeons still call themselves board-certified plastic surgeons when this isn't the case.

As someone who knows, firsthand, the tens of thousands of hours required to become a board-certified plastic surgeon, I'm shocked and disappointed at how many physicians call themselves "cosmetic surgeons," even though they are not board certified in surgery.

The bottom line is only a surgeon board certified in plastic surgery is qualified to perform breast augmentations. Just because other doctors are legally allowed to perform them doesn't mean they should. After all, they have not undergone the rigorous training, testing, and continuing education board-certified plastic surgeons have.

Board Certification Benefit: Research the Surgeon

One reliable and simple way to identify if your prospective surgeon is board certified in plastic surgery is to check with the American Board of Plastic Surgery, Inc. at www.abplsurg.org. Click on the "Is your surgeon certified?" link. You'll then be directed to a page where you can input your prospective surgeon's first and last name or the location of his or her practice.

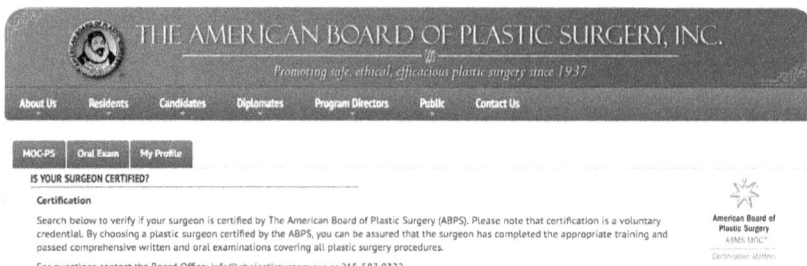

The site will indicate when the surgeon was certified and his or her current status with the board. This straightforward resource is one example demonstrating where board certification offers an unparalleled level of accountability, public exposure, and third-party oversight.

In addition, every state has its own medical board and state society for plastic surgery. For example, California's state society is the California Society of Plastic Surgeons (www.californiaplasticsurgeons.org). The Medical Board of California (www.mbc.ca.gov) also provides a powerful and reliable tool to research a prospective surgeon's track record.

For example, on the website of the Medical Board of California, when you click on "Verify a License," you'll find extensive information about the surgeon—specifically whether he or she has undergone any disciplinary action, which you'll see under the "Public Record Actions" section. If the doctor has engaged in negligent behavior, it will be reported there.

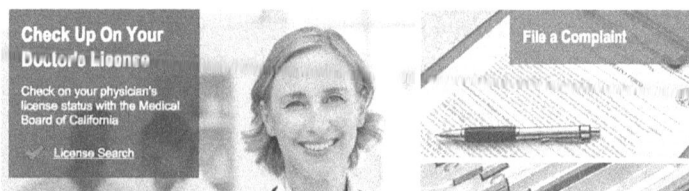

The Mission of the Medical Board of California

The mission of the Medical Board of California is to protect health care consumers through the proper licensing and regulation of physicians and surgeons and certain allied health care professions and through the vigorous, objective enforcement of the Medical Practice Act, and to promote access to quality medical care through the Board's licensing and regulatory functions.

Each state board is independent and maintains its own website. I encourage you to carefully review the state board website for your corresponding location when you're researching doctors.

What Are Hospital Privileges?

These are the authority and permission a doctor receives to provide patient care in a given hospital. To obtain privileges, doctors must submit an application that a governing board of the hospital will review. Surgeons must also undergo an additional screening process whereby they are directly observed performing surgery.

The more prestigious the hospital, the more difficult it is for a doctor to be granted privileges. In addition, a surgeon can be given privileges in multiple hospitals. Where the doctor has privileges is a reflection of his or her position in the medical community and status among his or her colleagues. Thus privileges are a demonstration of surgical excellence and medical community leadership.

For instance, I have privileges with Cedars Sinai in Los Angeles, which is one of the nation's top hospitals. While Los Angeles has one of the world's highest concentrations of plastic surgeons in the country, only a select number have been given privileges at Cedars Sinai.

On the doctor's site, he or she should state the location of hospital privileges. If they don't appear there, you should be able to quickly obtain the information by calling the doctor's office.

Memberships in Organizations

Just as board certification *is not* a prerequisite to practicing medicine, membership in professional organizations is optional as well.

Participation in **local**, **state**, and **national** groups is another indicator of a surgeon's relentless pursuit of staying on top of his or her surgical game. The following are examples of each:

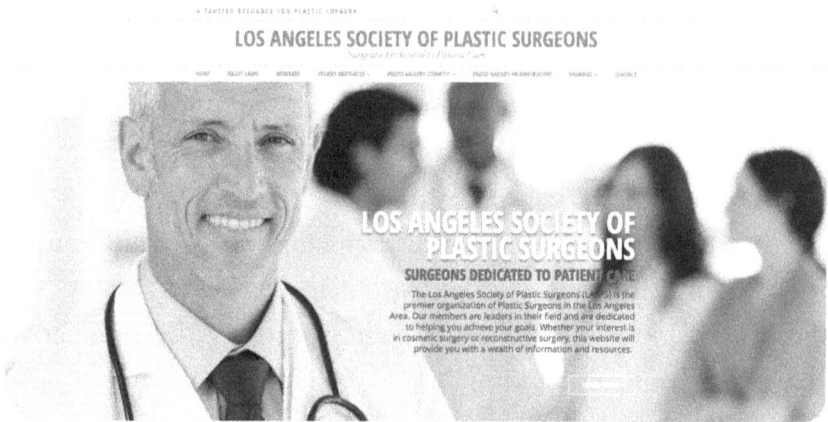

Local: For example, Los Angeles County's plastic surgery professional organization is the Los Angeles Society of Plastic Surgeons (LASPS).

State: Most states have their own plastic surgery professional organizations. For instance, in California it's called the California Society of Plastic Surgeons (CSPS).

National: There are two main groups: The American Society of Plastic Surgeons, Inc. (ASPS) and the American Society for Aesthetic Plastic Surgery (ASAPS).

Membership in one or more organizations demonstrates a doctor is staying at the forefront of his or her specialty, which means the surgeon is collaborating with colleagues, advocating on behalf of the profession, and teaching and learning breakthrough techniques. Membership also represents a commitment to lifelong learning, which includes participation in conferences and lectures.

In addition, taking on leadership positions within an organization reflects yet another level of professional dedication outside a doctor's individual practice. For example, I've been a member of the LASPS since I launched my Los Angeles practice. I was then recognized for my contributions to LASPS by being designated the organization's vice president.

Review Sites: Pluses and Minuses

From toppling oppressive political regimes to exposing a surgeon's sloppy patient service, social media has given anyone with an Internet connection unfettered ability to critique and assess all aspects of the world in which we live.

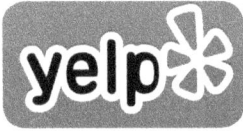

In regards to plastic surgery, the Internet has empowered patients with more information than ever before. It has enabled patients to report about their procedures, their recovery, and their experiences with a variety of plastic surgeons.

My practice has benefitted immensely from leveraging social media in its multiple and constantly changing forms. The positive reviews I've earned have motivated women across the country to schedule breast augmentations with me in my Beverly Hills office.

On the one hand, social media has strengths that are better than any other previous doctor-assessment tool. I believe rating-and-review sites and other forms of social media provide prospective breast augmentation patients with solid information that addresses *specific aspects* of a surgical procedure.

On the other hand, social media's strengths only apply to physician-to-patient interactions, individual patient experiences, and general trends that reflect the culture of a particular office. In other words, rating-and-review sites are a great way to measure the subjective aspects of the surgeon and his or her staff and to read anecdotal experiences patients have had.

In general, they are an effective tool to finding answers for the following subjective questions:

- Do the doctor and staff listen and communicate well?

- Are they warm, sincere, and know how to express genuine care and concern for their patients?

- Is their patient-service model consistent from the initial consultation to the post-op appointments?

But beyond these questions, social media's strengths unravel.

As you've read in this chapter, becoming a board-certified plastic surgeon is one of the world's toughest career paths. The technical and academic training requires tens of thousands of hours of intense study, relentless scrutiny by superiors, and surgical experience.

Thus, it's unreasonable to expect the same site that rates a local restaurant and nail salon to accurately assess a surgeon's skill. A doctor's expertise could never be reduced to a series of yellow stars. Allow me to illustrate:

Imagine someone you love must undergo life-or-death brain surgery. This person is incapacitated. As a result, you're left to find the best surgeon. In this made-up scenario, you must choose between one of two options:

1. A popular rating site you also use to find the city's best pizza and dry cleaner.

2. A site that describes the surgeon's educational background, licensing, years in practice, hospital privileges, membership in organizations, and professional history.

Clearly, you'd pick the second option to select the doctor who will save your loved one's life. But when it comes to breast augmentation, thousands of women across the country rely almost exclusively on rating-and-review sites whose metrics and formulas for selecting the so-called best surgeon are based on non-expert and completely subjective opinions and anecdotal evidence—a decidedly unscientific strategy to undergo a scientifically based procedure.

With that said, as much as I question the ability of a rating-and-review site to accurately assess the surgical performance of a physician, I still take the reviews and my overall rating seriously—mostly because my prospective patients count on them so much.

I've learned to embrace the sites because they have become a permanent part of the consumer landscape. In fact, patients regularly seek me out based solely on the solid series of reviews I've received.

No rating-and-review site can use its restaurant-rating formula as a substitute for the precise detail required to thoroughly and adequately assess a surgeon's skill.

Other Review Site Weaknesses

Just because a surgeon has a negative review, doesn't necessarily mean he or she is a bad doctor. This relates to a basic customer service truth: Satisfied customers rarely share about their positive experiences. If you're like me, you've probably received great service countless times throughout your life and you've gone about life as usual afterwards.

Unhappy customers, on the other hand, are more apt to share their negative experiences. Thus the rating-and-review sites are often complaint repositories, and their bias leans toward those who are searching for a forum to vent their dissatisfaction.

If, however, a surgeon has dozens of reviews and almost all of them are negative and nearly for the same reason, the ratings sites definitely provide valuable insight regarding broad trends within a practice.

Next, in your online search, you'll also encounter rating-and-review sites that exclusively focus on plastic surgery—no restaurants, bars, or plumbers included. While this seems compelling and credible, even these have questionable assessment metrics.

For example, many of these sites rank a particular doctor more favorably or higher based on how many advertising dollars he or she spends on their site.

One popular site ranks a surgeon based on how many public questions he or she answers. On this site, anyone can contribute a question. For instance, someone may ask, "What's the better implant: silicone or saline?" Surgeons who are members of the site input their answers. The more answers a doctor provides to questions submitted on the site, the higher his or her rating.

What I've found is most busy and successful surgeons do not have time to sit at a computer for hours every week fielding random questions entered by anyone who has Internet access and may or may not be serious about undergoing a breast augmentation.

In addition, for the sake of generating answers as quickly as possible, most doctors provide basic replies. In other words, their responses are ones any first-year medical school student can generate—in my opinion, this isn't the best reflection of a doctor's expertise.

So rating-and-review sites are fantastic ways to assess physician-to-patient interactions, individual patient experiences, and general trends that reflect the culture of a particular office—but not much else beyond this. In order to conduct thorough research, you must also identify a doctor's board certification, hospital privileges, and membership in professional organizations, as well as review his or her website.

The Surgeon's Own Website

When compared to other types of physicians, one advantage of researching plastic surgeons is many have individual websites that describe their practices. In fact, out of all board-certified doctors, plastic surgeons as a whole have always been at the forefront of the latest website developments.

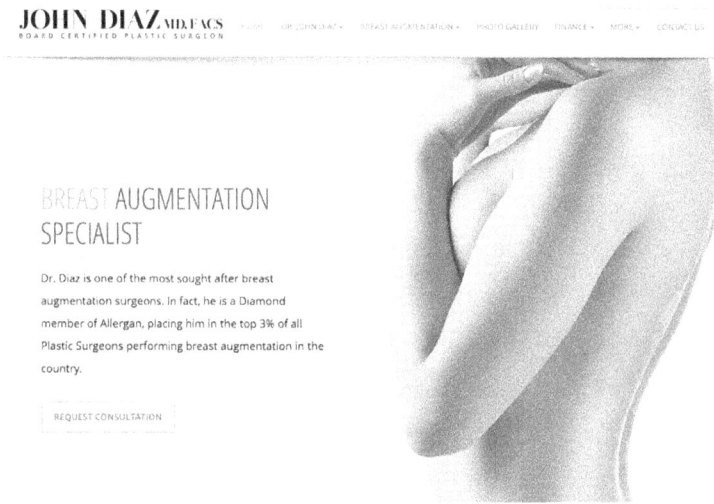

FIGURE 2.1. Website of Dr. John Diaz.

The following are three easy ways to perform a website assessment of a surgeon:

THE SITE'S LOOK AND FEEL

This reflects a site's visual design as well as the ease of navigating through it. Evaluating look and feel includes the following three sub-questions:

1. Is the site modern or dated?
The general appearance of the website will give you a sense of the doctor's present-day practice. If the site is full of current content

including up-to-date video presentations generated by the surgeon and recent patient before-and-after images, this signals the doctor is constantly staying up with trends. Overall, the doctor's site should show he or she is committed to remaining at the forefront of plastic surgery and educating the public.

The Internet is evolving and changing quickly. For instance, smart phones and tablets have altered how consumers interact with online content. A doctor should have two websites: one for computer screens and another for tablets and smartphones. By having both, this simple example demonstrates a doctor continually adjusts to meet the needs of his or her audience.

When a surgeon's site looks as if it was designed during the Windows 2000 era, is loaded with images that are equally as dated, and is nearly useless on a mobile device, this is clear sign the doctor's practice may be behind the times. In addition, old images make it difficult to assess how the surgeon works today.

2. Is the site organized or cluttered?
As the saying goes, "You never get a second chance to make a first impression." Websites are often the initial encounter prospective patients have with a surgeon.

One requirement of a great surgeon is an impeccable attention to detail. You want the site to show how the doctor runs his or her practice. A site should be easy to navigate on your computer or smartphone. It should be organized in a way that is intuitive. In other words, you're able to find the information you need quickly, such as doctor credentials, videos, and before-and-after images. If the site is disorganized and difficult to navigate, this reflects a doctor's failure to pay attention to his or her prospective patients' needs.

3. Is the site tasteful or flashy?

If a site demonstrates a doctor's personality and preferences, then you want one that reflects the type of surgeon you're searching for.

Some sites are sophisticated. The overall design emphasizes elegance and style. Meanwhile, other websites are full of garish breast images that appear all over the place—this may reflect how the surgeon perceives breast augmentation.

A surgeon's website is one of many tools you have to assess a doctor's expertise and skill. While in and of itself, a site is insufficient to make your final decision, its look and feel can reflect the surgeon's approach and philosophy regarding breast augmentation.

INFORMATION ON THE SITE

A surgeon's site should demonstrate his or her knowledge about breast augmentation. The information should be thorough *and* simple to understand. While doing one of these well is relatively easy, doing both skillfully requires expertise and an ability to communicate complicated concepts in a non-intimidating and straightforward fashion. If a doctor is a master online communicator, he or she will most likely be equally adept in person.

On the one hand, some doctors load their sites with breast augmentation information that is easily found anywhere on the web. Sometimes it seems as if these surgeons copied content from various sites and either paraphrased or unabashedly pasted the information directly onto theirs. This approach is somewhat sloppy, if not downright irresponsible.

On the other hand, custom-crafted, thoughtfully composed information a doctor has written will be instantly relevant to you. It will show the surgeon has worked with many patients, knows their greatest concerns, and is able to address them clearly. The more detailed and valuable the content he or she presents you, the more likely the surgeon has a true passion for breast augmentation and is eager to share his or her expertise and connect with you.

THE SITE'S PHOTOS AND VIDEOS

A large number of high-quality breast augmentation photos and videos represent a surgeon who is active and regularly performing breast augmentations. Lots of current before-and-after images will help you assess a surgeon's ability to create the results you seek.

Friends: The Good and the Bad

Referrals from friends and family can provide you unmatched and trusted insight into the breast augmentation results a doctor is able to deliver. They can motivate you to schedule an appointment right away, *or* they can be part of your process-of-elimination approach.

I've had many patients schedule surgeries with me because they loved the outcome of their friend's breast augmentation and they sought the experience my office provides to my patients.

I've also heard variations of the following: "My best friend's breasts are *huge*. With all due respect, I never want mine to ever look like those!"

The woman saying this often eliminated her best friend's surgeon from her list because she sought a different look. However, it may be that the friend specifically requested that size.

The bottom line is a friend's experience is a solid referral source, but it should play only one part in your multifaceted search strategy.

The First Phone Call: Your Top Five

Plastic surgery has taken center stage in popular culture. Talk show hosts *love* to dish on which celebrity has had work done. The latest photos of a star's post-op breasts instantly blow up on Instagram, Twitter, and Facebook. And whether online, on TV, or in print, the question, "Has she had breast augmentation?" creates instant and widespread buzz. But rather than focus on the superficial, this chapter has moved to the more significant and serious aspects of this life-changing surgical procedure and has provided comprehensive professional insight.

Once you've gone through the checklists and you've found surgeons who have met the criteria you've learned about, I recommend you narrow your list to approximately five doctors. If you have more than five, the time you spend scheduling appointments and attending them will overwhelm you. And the costs associated with surgeons who charge a consultation fee may add unexpected expense to your search. Smaller cities, in contrast, may not have as many plastic surgeons to choose from. In these cases, two to three surgeons may be enough.

When you have your top five surgeons, you're ready to call the office. The resulting conversation is an additional assessment tool. The communication style of the person on the other end of the call is a reflection of the one whose office you're calling—in other words, the surgeon. If the team member is polite, patient, and courteous, those same traits will most likely carry over in your first face-to-face meeting, which you'll learn about next. In chapter 3, we'll explore the introductory consultation.

Summary

- Always confirm that your doctor is a board-certified plastic surgeon.

- You should research where the doctor has hospital privileges and what organizations the doctor belongs to. This will give you an insight into the dedication the surgeon puts into his or her field.

- There are several great online resources to research doctors. These include the American Board of Plastic Surgery and your state's medical board.

- Rating-and-review sites, websites, blogs, and referrals from friends are helpful but limited in providing additional information about the surgeon's approach to patient care.

- After researching several doctors, narrow your list of potential surgeons to your top five choices. This will give you a variety of options without causing you to become overwhelmed.

After reading this chapter, you have the information necessary to find several excellent surgeons whom you will meet in person for your introductory consultation. In the next chapter, I will describe how to prepare for the consultation to make sure it is as productive and helpful as possible.

Breast Augmentation Myths

> The surgeon said he is a board-certified cosmetic surgeon. That means he is qualified to perform my surgery.

Only a board-certified *plastic surgeon* is qualified to perform a breast augmentation. Unfortunately, many unethical doctors imply they are plastic surgeons but are really not.

A doctor can be board certified, but that board certification may be in another specialty, such as ear, nose, and throat surgery or dermatology. These specialists do not have the appropriate training to perform a breast augmentation.

Also, just because someone says she is a cosmetic surgeon does not mean she has the training to perform cosmetic surgery. Cosmetic surgery is a generic term and is not regulated. Basically, anyone can call himself or herself a cosmetic surgeon.

The American Board of Medical Specialties (ABMS) carefully regulates the names given to various specialties. Plastic surgery, for example, is one of the approved specialties. Thus, if you want to make sure your doctor is qualified to perform your surgery, make sure he or she is board certified specifically in plastic surgery.

My surgeon was on a TV show. He must be good!

This may be one of the biggest myths in plastic surgery. Just because a surgeon is on a TV show does not mean he is a skilled surgeon. Sometimes he may be, but many times he isn't. I know because I have been on many TV programs over the years and saw firsthand what the process was like.

The priority of any TV show is its ratings. TV producers are under tremendous pressure to create programs that attract viewers and keep them interested. Thus, when producers are deciding whom to invite on to a show, they want to make sure the audience will be entertained, especially if it is a reality-based program.

Sometimes the surgeons are invited because they have a great reputation and come across well on TV. These are usually top surgeons who are leaders in their field—I like to think this was the reason I was invited to appear on as many programs as I have been!

But most of the time, surgeons are invited because they have over-the-top personalities or have some connection to a celebrity. This is how TV shows ensure they continue receiving high ratings. In this case, the surgeon is not invited because of his or her skill or experience.

So, if you like a surgeon you see on TV, remember that you still need to perform your research! If you follow the advice in this chapter, you will make sure that the surgeon is on TV because he is an amazing physician and not because he has a super-sized personality!

CHAPTER 3

THE
CONSULTATION

In this chapter, you'll learn:

- how to prepare for your first consultation;

- what to expect during your first consultation;

- common consultation myths and misconceptions.

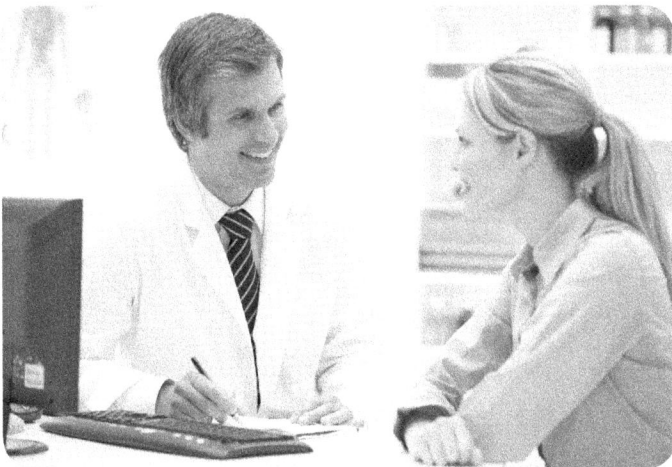

Real Conversations

Megan left her house thirty minutes before her plastic surgery consultation.

"Plenty of time to get to the doctor's," she told herself.

To her chagrin, a highway traffic accident followed by a series of surface-street red lights derailed her plan. By the time she pulled into the parking structure, she was already running fifteen minutes late for her 10:00 a.m. appointment.

Megan rushed to the front desk and checked in. The administrative assistant warmly greeted the harried patient and handed her a clipboard with forms to complete. After she filled out the paperwork, she was escorted to the examination room. It was 10:30 a.m., and another woman had arrived in the office.

"I'm here for my eleven o'clock appointment," the woman told the administrative assistant. "I know I'm a little early."

The woman's arrival signaled Megan's appointment with the doctor would promptly end at 11:00 a.m. Megan's hour-long consultation would now be reduced to thirty minutes at most.

On her smartphone, Megan had prepared a list of questions to ask the surgeon. But when she met with the doctor in the examination room, she knew she might not have time to refer to her list. In fact, after she had described the result she wanted and the doctor examined her, it was already time for the surgeon's next appointment. Sadly, Megan wasn't able to address any of her prepared questions. Worst of all, she didn't even get a chance to look at any of her implant options.

"If I'd only left the house earlier," she told herself.

The Consultation

Consultations vary widely from doctor to doctor. Some doctors provide an hour of their undivided attention to their patients.

Meanwhile, others have a staff member conduct most of the consultation. Then, ten minutes before the appointment's end, the doctor makes his or her appearance. In other words, there is no set formula all plastic surgeons follow.

With that said, most top surgeons make patient-education a top priority. They recognize the importance of effectively providing their insight and expertise using language their patients will understand.

Because of the wide variation among consultation styles, describing each would be an impossible task. Thus, in this chapter, I'll explain how I perform patient consultations. Throughout this chapter, I'll address you as if you were my patient. As a result, you'll gain insight into what a high-quality, patient-focused consultation looks like. If you're looking for the best consultation, you'll read about it in the following pages.

In addition, by following the structure of my patient consultation, you'll learn how to best prepare for your preliminary appointment, which is a meeting that will play an important role in your overall surgical experience.

Your Honorary Degree in Plastic Surgery

All plastic surgeons should be able to explain complex surgical procedures to their patients in a way that informs, rather than confuses. In fact, I often joke with my patients that by the end of their consultation, they'll know as much about breast augmentation as I do.

While there's no way a non-surgeon can fully understand everything a doctor who has completed medical school and residency and performed countless surgeries does, I tell my patients this because it reflects the priority I place on patient education and addressing a woman's most pressing concerns. The hour I spend with each prospective patient covers essential details, including implants, sizes, surgery, and recovery.

Arrive Early to Get the Most Out of Your Consultation

By giving yourself ample time prior to your consultation, you'll avoid what Megan experienced at the start of this chapter. Rather than have to rush through your appointment, you'll have plenty of time to complete paperwork, ask questions, and receive the information necessary to make informed and wise decisions.

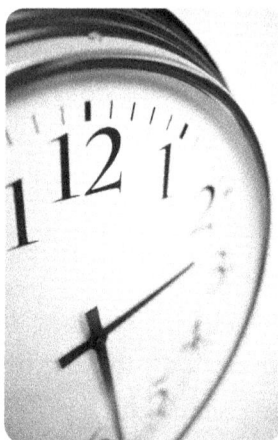

For example, plastic surgery offices throughout the country are frequently located in busy, high traffic areas. In my case, my practice is located in the heart of Beverly Hills. Throughout the day, the streets are packed with residents, tourists, and commuters. In this area, parking lots can quickly become full. Thus, finding a space can add a significant amount of time to your travel plans. And once you finally enter a surgeon's office, most will require you complete forms and questionnaires prior to your face-to-face meeting.

As a result, you want to make sure you allot enough time to drive, park, and fill out paperwork before your appointment to meet the doctor.

The forms and questionnaires you'll fill out prior to your face-to-face meeting typically ask for your date of birth, address, phone number, emergency contacts, procedures you're interested in, and an overview of your general health, as well as additional information.

In my practice, I've simplified the process by having forms and questionnaires on an iPad that patients receive when they arrive for the consultation—no clipboards loaded with cumbersome paperwork. Once you complete the necessary information, my staff escorts you to the consultation room.

The Face-to-Face Consultation: Do Your Homework

My assistant and I then join you in the consultation room. In order to create a customized and comprehensive surgical plan, I ask a series of questions that relate to your desired outcome. You should consider your answers before your appointment. By clearly articulating your objectives and concerns, you'll be better able to leverage my expertise.

In chapter 1, you learned about *Five Self-Assessment Questions:*

1. Why am I seeking breast augmentation?

2. Is this a good time for me to have surgery?

3. How much larger do I want my breasts to be?

4. What are my short-term and long-term goals?

5. What look do I want to achieve?

Questions three through five address the result you're seeking. Please refer to this section in chapter 1 for details on what to consider as you develop your answers. Your responses will put you in control of the consultation and help your surgeon provide the solutions you seek.

An Overview of the Physical Exam

Once I have the necessary information to determine the result you're looking for, you're ready for the physical exam. I take several detailed measurements of the chest and breast. These measurements allow me to narrow down the implant options that will give you the result you desire.

PHYSICAL EXAM: MEASUREMENTS

One of my responsibilities is to help you choose the right style and shape implant. The multiple measurements I take will provide the information I need to recommend implants that are proportional to your body and will provide the look you're seeking.

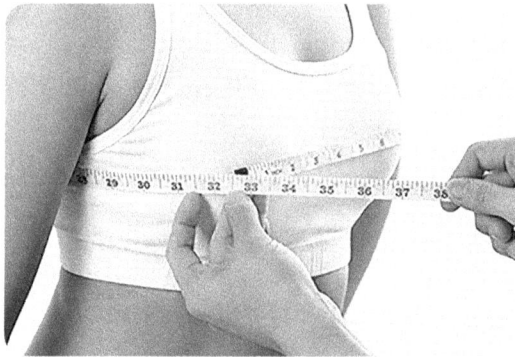

As you can imagine, the implant used will play an important role in the kind of result you'll achieve. Thus I recommend knowing some of your options *before* the consultation. Unfortunately, with thousands of implant options available and an abundance of misinformation, making informed decisions can be overwhelming. The good news is I've simplified your research. In chapter 4, you will receive an in-depth and easy-to-understand explanation of breast implants that will clear any confusion and misconceptions. For now, what you need to know is implants come in different shapes and sizes, and each one has a specific width.

This is why the breast *base diameter* (also called the *base width)* is one of the most important measurements. The base diameter refers to how wide each of your breasts is. It indicates how much space a breast has inside it to accommodate an implant. In other words, the width of the breast will determine the size and style of the implant.

In general*, an implant cannot be wider than your base diameter.* It must be as wide or less wide than your breast in order for your breast tissues to drape beautifully around it. If the implant is too wide, then it will not fit well. This is discussed in more detail in chapter 4.

Another measurement is the distance from the sternal notch to the nipple. The sternal notch is the dip at the bottom of your neck where your neck and chest meet. This measurement shows any differences between the right and left breasts.

The following are other measurements:

- Distance from the nipple to the inframammary fold, which is the bottom of the breast where it meets the chest skin

- The width of the areola

- The distance from the middle of the chest to each nipple

- How much the breast skin is able to stretch

The multiple measurements also identify any asymmetries in the size or shape of your breasts. I'll point these out during your exam. We need to consider asymmetries when developing your surgical plan. Some asymmetries require additional procedures or special techniques.

3D IMAGING: CUTTING-EDGE TECHNOLOGY PROVIDES UNPARALLELED INFORMATION

Once my assistant and I have recorded your measurements and you have narrowed your many implant options down to a few, we'll take detailed images of your breasts.

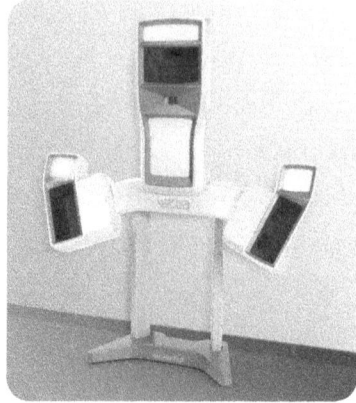

FIGURE 3.1.
The Vectra 3D imaging system.
This is a technologically
advanced imaging system.
It creates 3D images of your
chest and generates realistic
simulations of what you will
look like with any implant.

In my office, I use the *Vectra 3D imaging system* (see figure 3.1). Only a few surgeons in the world have this. The Vectra 3D camera takes multiple high-resolution photos of your breasts and converts them to three-dimensional images. The system then takes your breast images and provides simulations of what your breasts will look like with the implants you've selected. From there, you'll have ample time to review your results and decide which implants will best match the overall look you seek. Once you make your implant selection, I record your choice on your medical chart so it will be ready to order once you decide to undergo your augmentation.

The Vectra 3D imaging system provides you additional benefits. In chapter 5, I'll explain more about this breakthrough technology.

Once you have seen a realistic image of what your body will look like with the implant you've selected, you're ready to learn about the procedure itself.

OVER OR UNDER THE MUSCLE

During surgery, you have two options regarding where to place your implants: in the space located *below* or *above* the chest muscle. Each has advantages and disadvantages. I'll provide further insight into the pluses and minuses of your options in chapter 6.

INCISION LOCATION: MULTIPLE OPTIONS

During surgery, you have multiple options regarding the insertion point of your implants. They can be inserted through the bellybutton, the underarm, the areola, or the crease at the bottom of the breast. Each has its advantages and disadvantages. I'll provide further insight into the pluses and minuses of your options in chapter 7.

WHAT HAPPENS ON THE SURGERY DAY

During this part of the consultation, I explain, step by step, what you should expect on your surgery day. I'll provide detailed information regarding what will take place from the moment you arrive for your surgery appointment to when you leave my surgical center.

No doubt, you'll have a lot of information to keep track of. Thankfully, you won't have to remember it all. In chapter 10, we'll cover key details you'll need to know.

THE RECOVERY: A DETAILED DESCRIPTION

The last part of the consultation will review what your recovery will be like. In chapter 11, I'll describe how your recovery will progress from the moment we complete your procedure to what will take place in the days, weeks, and months ahead. I'll also guide you through how to plan appropriately for life after your breast augmentation.

After the Consultation

The entire consultation takes about an hour. Once we've completed the physical exam, viewed 3D images, and discussed implant and incision placement, surgery, and recovery, you're then ready to meet with my patient coordinator.

The patient coordinator will provide details regarding how to schedule your surgery and what the associated costs will be.

At this point, if you've done your homework by consulting with other surgeons and you've determined which doctor you'll work with, you're ready to schedule your breast augmentation. In my office's case, my patient coordinator then will set your surgery date and guide you through the steps you'll need to take in order to ensure your breast augmentation day runs as smoothly as possible.

Summary

- Make sure to arrive early for your consultation.

- Take time to think about your answers to the Five Self-Assessment Questions. This will help you better communicate your goals to the surgeon.

- A high-quality consultation, such as the kind I conduct, should include a conversation about your goals, detailed measurements, a discussion of implant options, 3D simulations, and a review of the surgery and recovery process.

Now that you've received an overview of what a high-quality consultation looks like, you're ready to dive deeper into the process. In the next chapter, I'll describe everything you need to know about the implants themselves.

Breast Augmentation Myths

Consultations with a plastic surgeon are free.

Although some consultations are free, most top plastic surgeons include a fee for their initial consultation. This is an investment in the doctor's expertise and time he or she will spend with you. Fortunately, most offices will apply the consultation fee to the cost of the surgery. The investment in a surgeon with a great reputation is well worth the amount you pay.

The plastic surgeon won't spend a lot of time with me during the consultation.

In my practice I work every day to expose the fallacy of this myth. I believe that breast augmentation is an incredibly important decision in your life. As such, you deserve to have this procedure and all of its options carefully explained to you. Unfortunately, most plastic surgeons do not spend enough time with patients during the consultation. I, on the other hand, make sure to spend as much time as I can with you to review all the information you need to know and to answer all your questions.

CHAPTER 4

IMPLANTS

In this chapter, you'll learn:

- the differences between saline, silicone, and shaped implants;

- the differences between low, moderate, moderate-plus, high, and extra-high profile implants;

- how shaped implants differ from round implants;

- how implant size or volume is measured.

Real Conversations

Stephanie was thrilled that the day of her initial consultation with Dr. Kramer had finally arrived. Although she had intended to research about implants before her appointment, she neglected to do so.

At 11:00 a.m., Stephanie arrived at Dr. Kramer's office. The receptionist checked her in and escorted Stephanie to the consultation room. Shortly after, Dr. Kramer introduced himself. During their talk, the surgeon described the various types of implants available. After trying to keep track of a few of them, she noticed her palms grew sweaty. "So many options, and I don't really know what he's talking about," she told herself as she attempted to follow his descriptions.

Dr. Kramer then made his implant recommendation. By this point, Stephanie suffered from information overload and struggled to understand the specific reasons why he recommended the particular implant.

After her appointment, Stephanie reached her car and slumped in the driver's seat. "I've left the consultation more confused than when I arrived," she said to herself. She wished she had done preliminary research beforehand.

So Many Implant Choices!

Quick question: How many different types of implants do you think there are?

Believe it or not, you'll find over two thousand options! This high number is largely a result of the multiple combinations of fills, shapes, styles, and textures on the market (you'll learn about each of these in this chapter). And every implant option has its own particular advantages and disadvantages.

No doubt, reviewing thousands of implants can be exhausting, and deciding which implant is best for you can be overwhelming. The good news is I've simplified your search. In this chapter, I've organized your implant options in a straightforward and easy-to-understand way. Within these pages, you'll learn everything you need to know about breast implants. After reading this chapter, you'll be an implant pro You'll have the resources to narrow down the type of implant that matches the result you seek.

The Anatomy of an Implant

In this section, I'll explain the different implant features. By understanding an implant's structure, you'll have the information necessary to work with your surgeon to select the best implant for you.

Implants: The Shell and Surface Texture

First, let's begin with the implant's outer layer. No matter the type, all implants have a covering called a **shell**. This is a thin material that surrounds the implant. It provides a barrier between whatever is inside and outside the implant.

Whether you're referring to a saline or silicone implant, *all shells are made of silicone.* This is because silicone has particular qualities that make it an effective outer layer: It's thin, strong, and impermeable. So, although the shell is barely noticeable, it provides a long-lasting barrier to prevent anything leaking into or out of it.

Next, there are two types of implant surface textures: **smooth surface** and **textured surface** (see figure 4.1).

FIGURE 4.1. Smooth and textured implants.
The smooth surface implant is in the back;
the textured surface implant is in the front.

Smooth-surface implants are by far the most common. Their surface feels slick, similar to that of a balloon. On the other hand, textured implants have a rougher surface comprising microscopic bumps. Many people describe a textured-surface implant as feeling like velvet.

The main purpose of the microscopic bumps in textured-surface implants is to reduce the risk of **capsular contracture**. Capsular contracture is hardening of the scar around a breast implant. When women develop this, the breasts feel firmer. Whether textured-surface implants actually decrease capsular contracture is debatable: Some studies have shown that they reduce the risk of capsular contracture, while other studies have shown they do not. Thus, deciding between smooth- and textured-surface implants comes down to reviewing other aspects.

Textured-surface implants can create a stronger attachment to the underside of the breast skin, resulting in mild but visible irregularities such as dimpling on the skin's surface. Given this rare but potential risk and the fact that textured-surface implants haven't been conclusively shown to decrease capsular contracture, they are less commonly used than smooth-surface implants.

FILL: SALINE AND SILICONE

"Dr. Diaz, should I get saline or silicone implants?" a patient will ask me. This is by far the most common question I receive. In this section, we'll explore the advantages and disadvantages of each.

First, allow me to clarify what these patients are asking. Beneath the implant's smooth or textured surface is the **fill**, which is the material inside the implant itself. You have two fill options: saline (salt water) or silicone. (As you've learned, whether they're called saline or silicone implants, their shell is always silicone.)

Saline Fill: Overview

Saline implants arrive at your surgeon's office unfilled in a sterile package (see figure 4.2). During surgery, the doctor connects a filling tube to the implant. The implant is then filled with a sterile saltwater solution. This solution is similar to the fluid that makes up most of the human body. Once the saline implant is filled to the chosen size, the doctor then removes the tube and seals the implant's opening.

FIGURE 4.2. A saline implant. The valve located at the top of the implant allows it to be filled with saline during surgery."

SALINE FILL: PLUSES AND MINUSES

Pluses: Given that saline implants are filled with a saltwater solution, many patients believe saline implants must be safer to use than silicone implants. You will find a lot of comments supporting this on informal blogs and chat rooms.

However, numerous scientific studies conducted over the past twenty years all prove silicone implants are just as safe as their saline counterparts. Despite the overwhelming evidence supporting the safety of silicone implants, however, a small number of women still simply feel more comfortable knowing their implants are filled with saline.

One possible advantage of saline implants is a surgeon can easily adjust their size. As a result, the doctor has slightly more flexibility in sizing during the procedure itself. With that said, silicone implants come in a wide variety of sizes. Thus most surgeons do not consider saline's adjustability a significant advantage.

Another plus for many patients is saline implants are less expensive than silicone implants. Therefore, the cost of surgery using saline implants may be more affordable.

Minuses: Saline implants tend to feel firmer than silicone implants. This firmness may seem less natural when compared to silicone implants.

Saline implants also have a higher risk of **rippling** than silicone implants. Rippling is when the implant's edges can be seen or felt. This is usually more noticeable along the bottom and the side of the breasts. And textured saline implants may demonstrate the rippling effect even more.

Silicone Fill: Overview

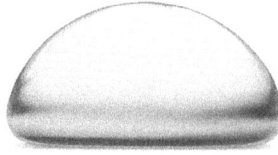

FIGURE 4.3. A silicone implant.

Silicone implants are filled with sterile, medical-grade silicone gel. (See figure 4.3.) Compared to today's silicone implants, previous ones were filled with a more liquid form of silicone and had a weaker shell. This made them prone to breaking or rupturing, which made the implants more difficult to remove and for breasts to be re-operated on. In order to remedy these drawbacks, silicone implant manufacturers worked painstakingly to improve silicone implant safety and reliability.

The latest generation of silicone implants has a much stronger outer shell and a thicker form of silicone gel inside. This gel is highly cohesive, which means it is very thick and maintains its shape even when the implant shell is compromised. Therefore, in the unlikely event a silicone implant breaks or ruptures, the gel inside should stay securely in place. (See figure 4.4.)

Another version of silicone implant is called "highly cohesive, shaped silicone gel implant." Quite a mouthful, isn't it? It is commonly referred to as a "shaped anatomic" or "gummy bear" implant. The fill of shaped anatomic implants consists of an even thicker version of

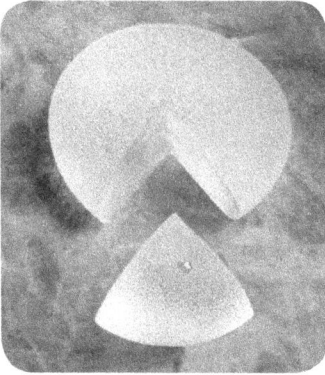

FIGURE 4.4.
This silicone implant has been cut. Note the consistency of the gel inside the implant. It is a thick gel that does not leak out of the implant.

silicone than regular silicone implants. This thicker version of silicone gel helps maintain the unique shape of the "gummy bear" implant. This shape will be discussed in more detail later in the chapter.

SILICONE FILL: PLUSES AND MINUS

Pluses: Silicone implants typically feel softer and more natural than saline implants. In fact, most patients agree that silicone implants feel just like natural breasts.

Another advantage of silicone implants is they show significantly less rippling than saline implants. This is a major benefit because most women find rippling troublesome and unsightly.

When it comes to safety, previous silicone implants had received widespread media coverage for being dangerous. But multiple scientific studies have proven this common misconception wrong. As you learned earlier, research shows silicone implants are *just as safe* as saline implants.

Minus: Overall, silicone implants are more expensive than saline implants. Thus the cost of surgery may be higher when compared to saline implants.

Style

Saline and silicone implants are categorized according to their **style.** Although style is the term implant manufacturers use, it actually refers to the implant's shape. I'll use both terms interchangeably throughout this book.

Implants come in a variety of shapes, and each one achieves a slightly different result. These are the general categories of shapes:

- Low profile (may also be called "moderate profile")

- Moderate-plus profile

- High profiles (includes high and extra high profiles)

- Shaped-anatomic profile (also called "gummy bear")

The following image shows the shapes of the three following implant categories: low, moderate-plus, and high-profile shapes. (See figure 4.5.)

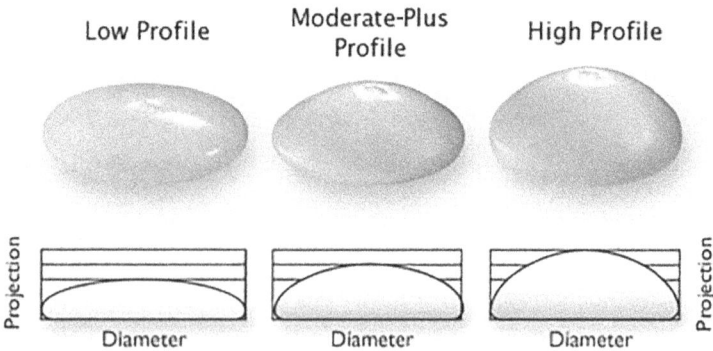

FIGURE 4.5. The shapes of low, moderate-plus, and high profile implants.

Shape Measurements

An implant's particular shape is a combination of the following:

- Diameter (or width)—how wide it is

- Height—how tall it is

- Projection—how much it "sticks out" from the chest

- Volume—its size or how much saline it holds

Let's explore each.

DIAMETER

The implant's diameter refers to how wide the implant is when viewed from the front. This is measured in centimeters.

HEIGHT

This refers to how tall the implant is from the bottom to the top of the breast. Shaped, or "gummy bear," implants have three height options:

- Full height, abbreviated as F

- Moderate height, abbreviated as M

- Low height, abbreviated as L

PROJECTION

This refers to how much the implant "sticks-out" from your chest. Shaped implants have four projection options:

- Low projection, abbreviated as L

- Moderate projection, abbreviated as M

- Full projection, abbreviated as F

- Extra-full projection, abbreviated as X

VOLUME

The final way to characterize implants is by their volume. The volume refers to how much saline or silicone the implant contains. Volume is measured in cubic centimeters. One cubic centimeter (cc) equals one milliliter (ml). One cc (1 ml) is about one-fifth of a teaspoon.

Volume and Cup Size

Implants do not come in cup sizes because the amount of cubic centimeters (cc) required to create a specific cup size will depend on multiple factors. These include your height and weight, how much breast tissue you have, the width of each of your breasts, the style or shape of implant you choose, and the brand and style of bra you prefer. This is why there is no way to guarantee how many cc you'll need in order to have a certain cup-size bra.

Although there is no direct cc to cup-size formula, the following are general guidelines:

- 200 to 300 cc will result in a B cup for most women

- 300 to 400 cc will result in a regular C to a full C cup for most women

- 400 to 450 cc will result in a D cup for most women

- 450 cc and up will likely result in a DD cup for most women

Keep in mind these are only estimates. The role of a detailed and thorough consultation is to provide you specific volume recommendations based on your body type and preferences.

Volume and Saline Fill

As you learned, saline implants come unfilled in a sterile package. During the surgery itself, they are filled with saline.

Each implant is designed to hold a certain range of saline solution. The lowest volume it can hold is called the "minimal-fill." The largest volume it can hold is called the "maximal-fill." For example, a 350 cc saline implant can be filled from a minimal fill of 350 cc to maximal fill of 380 cc. The range for any given saline implant from its minimal to maximal fill is usually around 30 cc. Differences in volume less than 20 cc to 30 cc are barely visible.

When a 350 cc implant is filled with 350 cc of saline, the implant is called "minimally filled." At 380 cc, it's called "maximally filled." Saline implants *are not designed to be filled less than their minimal fill or more than their maximal fill.* This is because filling saline implants below or above their specific ranges changes their dynamics and increases the likelihood of rupture.

Volume and Silicone Fill

All silicone implants come prefilled with a certain amount of cc. Unlike saline implants, the volume cannot be adjusted or changed during surgery because the size of a given style of silicone implant is preset. Silicone implants increase or decrease in size in increments of about 20 to 25 cc. This is because it is almost impossible to see any difference in size if there is less than a 20 to 25 cc difference in volume.

Shape: Bringing All the Measurements Together

Now that you've learned about an implant's individual measure-ments (diameter, height, projection, and volume), let's see how they come together to create multiple shapes. (See figure 4.6.)

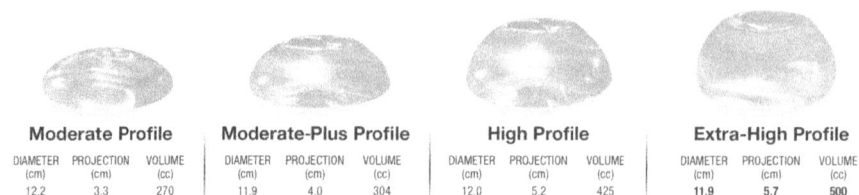

Moderate Profile			Moderate-Plus Profile			High Profile			Extra-High Profile		
DIAMETER (cm)	PROJECTION (cm)	VOLUME (cc)	DIAMETER (cm)	PROJECTION (cm)	VOLUME (cc)	DIAMETER (cm)	PROJECTION (cm)	VOLUME (cc)	DIAMETER (cm)	PROJECTION (cm)	VOLUME (cc)
12.2	3.3	270	11.9	4.0	304	12.0	5.2	425	11.9	5.7	500

FIGURE 4.6. The relationship between diameter, projection, and volume of moderate (low), moderate-plus, high, and extra-high profile implants.

If you look at the first column for each implant above, you'll notice the diameters of the implants are quite close in centimeters: 12.2, 11.9, 12.0, and 11.9 centimeters, respectively. So they vary by only about 0.3 centimeters (3 millimeters), which is negligible. This means these four implants are basically the same width.

Although the implants are all nearly the same width, you proba-bly noticed they look different from one another. So what accounts for the contrasting appearances?

It's their projection. If you look at the other two columns under each picture, you'll see measurements listed for the implant's projec-tion and volume. Notice that as the profile increases from moderate to extra-high, the projection increases (and, for the most part, the width stays the same).

As the projection increases, the space inside the implant also increases, and the implant is able to hold more saline or silicone. In fact, despite nearly identical widths, the volume increases from 270 cc for the low (or moderate) profile implant to 500 cc for the extra-high profile implant. You may have also noticed the implant becomes much rounder as the profile increases.

In summary, the higher the implant's profile, the rounder it becomes and the more volume it can hold. Why is this important? Because each of these implants will create a slightly different result. In the next section, I've summarized the features of the different implant shapes:

LOW PROFILE

- Also called "moderate profile"

- Tends to create a wider breast with a small amount of projection

- Is rarely used because most women want their implants to provide a greater projection of their breasts

MODERATE-PLUS PROFILE

- Tends to create some roundness at the top of the breasts, but most of the fullness is at the bottom (figure 4.7)

- Is a very popular implant

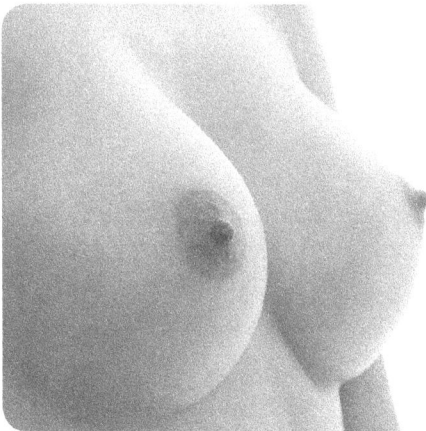

FIGURE 4.7. An example of the kind of shape a moderate-plus profile implant is designed to achieve. (This is a model and not a patient.)

HIGH PROFILE

- Tends to create more fullness over the top of the breasts (figure 4.8)

- Works especially well if you're seeking maximum size and roundness

- Is less popular than the moderate-plus profile implant because most women prefer having less fullness over the top of their breasts

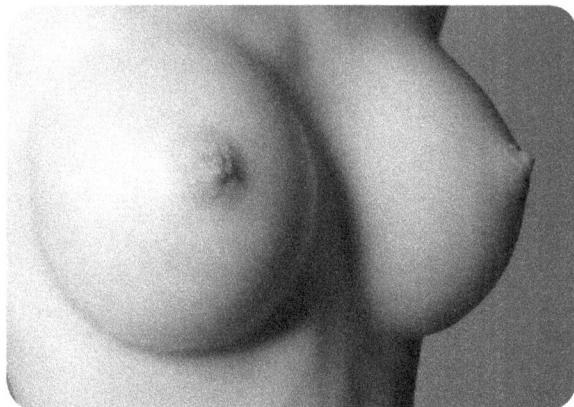

FIGURE 4.8. An example of the kind of shape a high-profile implant is designed to achieve. (This is a model and not a patient.)

EXTRA-HIGH PROFILE

- Tends to create exaggerated fullness over the top of the breasts

- Causes pressure on the breast skin and the rib cage below the muscle

- Can cause long-term ribcage and breast skin problems so it is not routinely recommended

SHAPED ANATOMIC PROFILE
(ALSO CALLED "GUMMY BEAR")

- Mimics the anatomy of a beautiful and natural female breast

- Creates a "tear drop" shape with the majority of the fullness located at the bottom of the breast (figures 4.9 and 4.10)

FIGURE 4.9. A shaped anatomic implant.

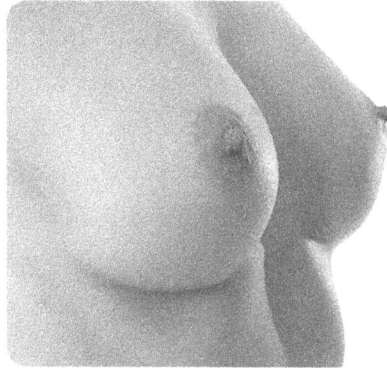

FIGURE 4.10. An example of the kind of result a shaped, anatomic implant is designed to achieve. (This is a model and not a patient.)

- Has a textured surface

- Is available with saline fill, but the vast majority are silicone filled

- Must be positioned perfectly inside the breast because of its special shape

- Is less commonly used than the moderate-plus profile because it was introduced more recently but is becoming more popular every year

MORE ABOUT THE SHAPED ANATOMIC PROFILE

Shaped anatomic profile implants come in a wide range of shapes and sizes. This provides the surgeon significant control over the final outcome and yields a result tailored to your body and preferences.

These implants must be positioned perfectly inside the breast. This is because, unlike other implants, shaped profile implants will look different depending on how they are positioned. If the shaped profile implant rotates after surgery, it will distort the appearance of the breast. This is one risk associated with these implants. In order to prevent distortion, the surgeon must make sure the implants are perfectly positioned. Also, all shaped implants have a textured surface to make it harder for them to slide around or rotate after surgery. Fortunately, the risk of this happening is exceedingly rare.

Shaped anatomic profile implants come in a wide range of options. In addition to the shapes and sizes, they can also vary in their height and projection. This provides the surgeon significant control over the final outcome and provides you with a result tailored to your body and preferences. The images below show the differences between shaped anatomic profiles (see figures 4.11 and 4.12).

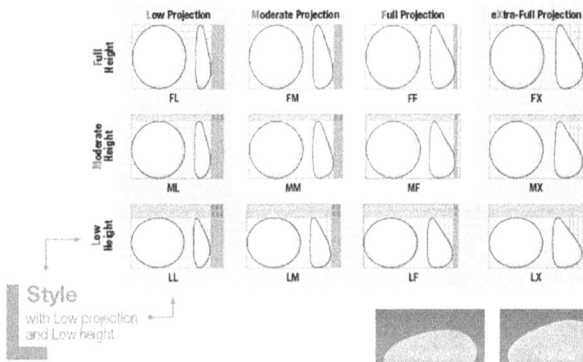

FIGURE 4.11. An illustration of all the options in projection and height for shaped, anatomic implants.

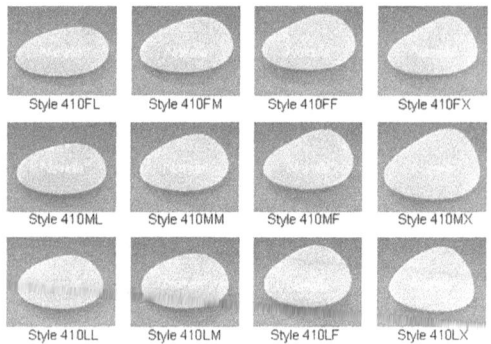

FIGURE 4.12. Pictures of the different projection and height options for shaped, anatomic implants.

During an in-depth consultation, your doctor should review all your implant style options.

Summary

- All implants have an outer covering, or shell, made of a thin layer of silicone.

- The surface of the implant can be smooth or textured.

- Implants are filled with either saline (salt water) or medical-grade pure silicone gel.

- Implants come in a variety of styles or shapes. These include low profile, moderate-plus profile, high profile, and extra-high profile.

- Implants also come in a shaped anatomic profile (commonly referred to as the "gummy bear" implant).

- Each style or shape is designed to create a specific result.

- Implants also come in a range of volumes, measured in cc.

- Each implant has its own specific advantages and disadvantages. You and your surgeon should work closely together to develop a surgical plan that considers all your options and addresses your needs.

In addition to reviewing implant style options, your surgeon should describe how many cc your implants will require in order to achieve your desired result. In addition, some doctors use 3D imaging to show you what each implant size will look like on your particular body. You'll learn more about how to select a size and the role of 3D imaging in the next chapter.

Breast Augmentation Myths

Saline implants are safer than silicone implants.

No evidence suggests that saline (saltwater) implants are any safer than the silicone implants available today. In fact, numerous studies have explored whether or not silicone implants increase the chance of complications or side effects after surgery. All these studies have proven that silicone implants are equally as safe as saline ones.

I have to replace implants (either silicone or saline) after ten years.

No. The misconception that you have to replace your implants after a decade has been widely reported in the media and popular culture.

This widespread myth was a result of misinterpreting research that focused on women undergoing breast augmentation. In one study, a group comprising hundreds of women was followed for over ten years after their breast augmentation.

The study showed that the vast majority of women who received breast implants did, indeed, have them changed within a decade. But closer analysis of the data revealed the true reasons why. The majority of the woman who were included in the study were in their early twenties. Over the course of ten years, many of these women became pregnant, had children, and breastfed.

As a result, in the ten years that followed the test group's breast augmentations, the women's breasts underwent the normal changes that any female's breasts would have. Some women developed sagging of the breasts. Other women felt that their breasts became either too small or too large after pregnancy. Thus, many of them had surgery for the same reasons anyone seeks surgery. Some wanted larger implants, others sought new implants and a breast lift, and some wanted to change their saline implants to silicone implants. This means that many of the women replaced their implants because they wanted to—not because they had to.

No doubt, some of the women in the study did change their implants because of complications such as capsular contracture or dissatisfaction with their initial result. But the majority replaced their implants voluntarily.

While the media focused on the women in the study who had changed their implants within ten years, the media frequently failed to describe the real reasons why. The fact is the current forms of implants are safe and you will only need to replace them if you have a complication or if you want to change them for other reasons.

If I get silicone implants, I have to have an MRI done every two years.

No. The older style of silicone implants had a weak shell and a more liquid form of silicone inside compared with today's silicone implants. This increased the likelihood that they could break open or rupture. In the past, if a silicone implant did break open, the silicone would spill out and the breast would deflate.

As a result, it was relatively easy to tell if an old silicone implant had ruptured because the breast shape would change. But new silicone implants have a stronger outer covering and a thick silicone gel inside.

In fact, nowadays, it's extremely rare for silicone implants to rupture. But even if they do, the silicone stays inside the implant. Thus, if the current version of silicone implants were to rupture, you may not even notice; the breast shape would remain the same because the silicone gel would not leak out of the implant.

So barring surgery, the only way to reliably know if a silicone implant has ruptured is to obtain an MRI of the breasts. This is the reason why the FDA and implant manufacturers recommend an MRI every two years. In other words, the MRI's purpose is to diagnose if a rupture is present.

But this is only a recommendation. It is not mandatory. So the vast majority of women who obtain an MRI will not have evidence of rupture. Furthermore, even if the MRI did show a rupture, it is unlikely it would be associated with any changes in the shape or feel of the breast. So even if the implants were ruptured, no treatment may be necessary.

In summary, yes, both the FDA and the silicone-implant manufacturers recommend you obtain an MRI of the breasts every two years. But no, this is not mandatory.

CHAPTER 5

CHOOSING YOUR IMPLANT SIZE

In this chapter, you'll learn:

- how implant sizes are determined;

- approaches to selecting your implant size;

- what 3D imaging is.

Real Conversations

Before she met with Dr. Brennan, Jennifer had researched implants on her own and thought she already knew the size she wanted. During the consultation, she was shown what seemed like a million before-and-after breast augmentation photos. Now, after reviewing the near-endless series of patient images, she was no longer sure what size she wanted.

"The same implant looks totally different on two different people," she told herself as she scanned the images. "Now, I'm not sure

A COMPREHENSIVE GUIDE TO BREAST AUGMENTATION

if the size I wanted before will look good on me."

Given her uncertainty, she was worried she would pick the wrong implant. She wished there was a better way to decide.

Introduction

In the previous chapter, you learned about the different types of implants available to you, their advantages and disadvantages, and how they are measured. Armed with this information, you're more prepared than ever to select the implant type that best matches the outcome you seek.

Once you've decided your implant type, the next step is to pick your implant size. In my experience meeting patients who visit my office from around the world, *this is consistently the most difficult decision for women to make;* they have multiple options and have to commit to one size. A feeling of information overload is common. Fortunately, this chapter will add clarity to your search. You'll learn the essential information you need to determine the size that's right for you.

CC vs. Cup Size: How Implant Sizes Work

My patients are often surprised when I tell them that implants aren't available by cup size. In other words, you won't find a B-cup implant, C-cup implant, and so on. In this section, you'll learn why.

Previously, I described that the fill of an implant, whether saline or silicone, is measured in cubic centimeters, abbreviated as cc. This is a scientific way to measure volume, which is the amount of fluid your implant contains. One cubic centimeter (1 cc) is equal to one milliliter (ml), which is equal to about ¼ teaspoon. So one cc is a very small amount! (See figures 5.1 and 5.2.) The advantage of measuring implants by cc is it's a uniform unit of volume. In other words, one cc is the same, no matter what type of implant you choose.

Thus the measurement-by-cc approach means implant volumes

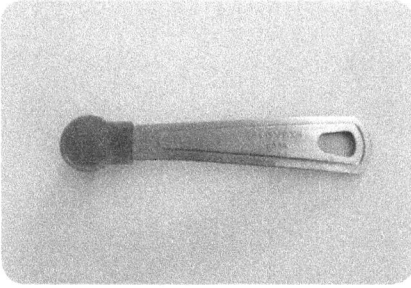

FIGURE 5.1.
One fourth of a teaspoon.
This is approximately 1 cc.

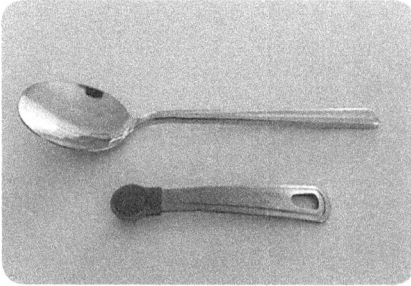

FIGURE 5.2.
One cc compared to
an average spoon.

are consistent across manufacturers. Contrast this uniformity with cup sizes. Although the letters are uniform—A, B, C, D—what they actually represent varies from bra brand to bra brand. For instance, you could be one cup size according to one bra maker and another cup size according to another bra maker. Even within one bra manufacturer, cup sizes can vary, depending on the bra style. Thus, there is no reliable cup-size standard.

To make matters even more confusing, one implant size can yield different cup sizes for different women, even if they all wear the same bra style within the same bra company. For example, an implant that measures 300 cc may result in a B cup for one woman, a C cup for another woman, and a D cup for yet another woman.

"How is this possible?" you may ask. The answer lies in the multiple factors that play a role in your final cup size, such as the implant itself, how much breast tissue you have before surgery, your height, how much you weigh, and the brand of bra you wear. Thus, it is impossible to guarantee a specific cup size for any implant.

Although you have no reliable way to match an implant's cc with a bra's cup size, the following are general guidelines, which you learned about previously:

- 200 to 300 cc will result in a B cup for most women (see figure 5.3)

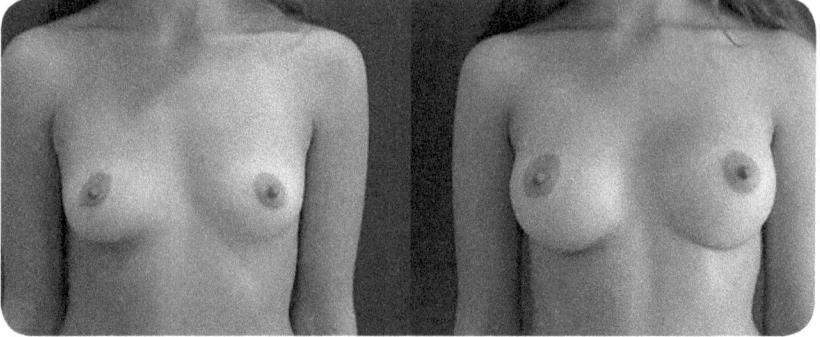

FIGURE 5.3. This patient had a 265 cc implant inserted. She increased from an A cup to a full B cup.

- 300 to 400 cc will result in a regular C to a full C cup for most women (see figure 5.4)

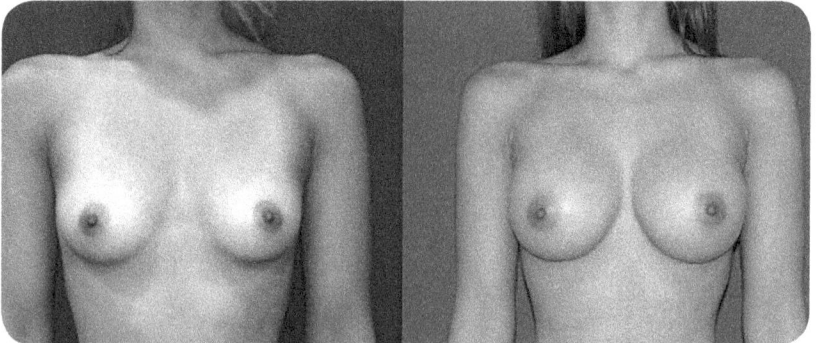

FIGURE 5.4. This patient had a 360 cc implant inserted. She increased from an A cup to a full C cup.

- 400 to 450 cc will result in a D cup for most women (see figure 5.5)

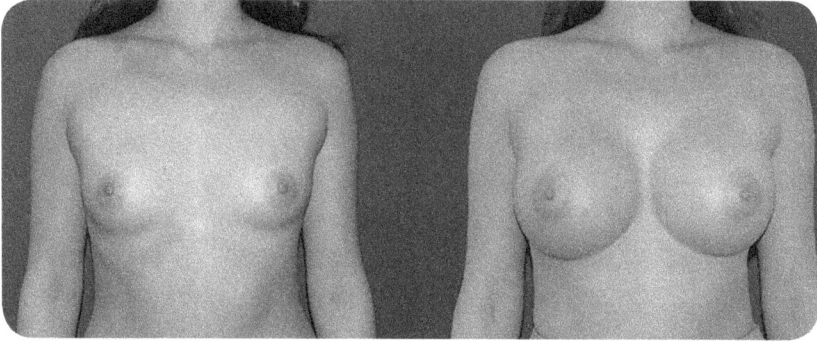

FIGURE 5.5. This patient had a 400 cc implant inserted. She increased from an A cup to a D cup.

- 450 cc and up will likely result in a DD cup for most women

Remember, these are only estimates. You'll need a thorough consultation with your surgeon in order to determine the implant size that best meets your needs.

What Size Is Right for You?

Experience has taught me that most patients have an image in their mind of the outcome they seek after surgery. It could be a picture of a model or celebrity they admire. Or it may be how the patient appears in a certain padded bra or dress.

If you can relate to what I've described, the challenge is to accurately express to your doctor what the image in your mind looks like, so he or she understands precisely what you seek.

Questions to Ask Yourself

A simple way to have a productive and informed discussion with your surgeon regarding implant size is to answer the following questions ahead of your appointment:

1. Overall, what do I want my breasts to look like?

2. Do I seek roundness or a more natural teardrop shape?

3. Do I want full and voluptuous or more conservative-looking breasts?

4. Do I seek a B, C, D, or DD cup size?

Next, write down your answers. Then bring your responses to your consultation. They will provide your surgeon important background information to help you meet your breast augmentation goals.

Collect Photos

Prior to an appointment, I tell my patients to collect photos that reflect breast images that appeal to them. These can be from a website, a magazine, or an Internet search. A popular strategy is to use pictures of celebrities (see figures 5.6, 5.7, and 5.8). During our consultation, my patients will show me photos saved on their mobile devices or images they've brought with them. Similarly, I suggest you compile photos as well.

Patients often bring pictures of lingerie models as examples of results they like. One thing to keep in mind when you look at these images is that the lingerie often pushes the breasts together, making the breasts appear larger and closer together than they really are. In addition, the models often use their arms to push the breasts even closer together, further enhancing the size and cleavage (see figure 5.9). Thus, the breasts of lingerie models might not actually be as large as they look.

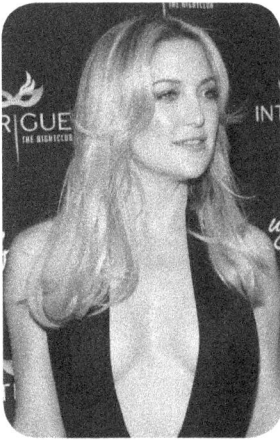

FIGURE 5.6. Kate Hudson. She is estimated to have B cup breasts. (Kate Hudson is not a patient, and I have never treated her.)

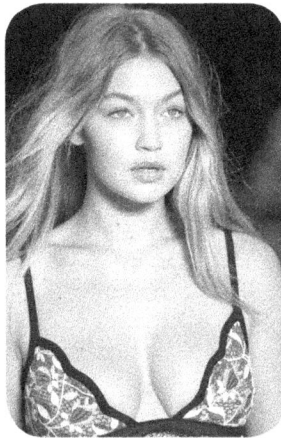

FIGURE 5.7 Gigi Hadid. Estimated to have C cup breasts. (Gigi Hadid is not a patient, and I have never treated her.)

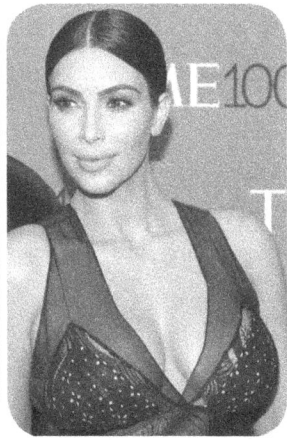

FIGURE 5.8 Kim Kardashian. Estimated to have full D cup breasts. (Kim Kardashian is not a patient, and I have never treated her.)

Providing your surgeon images will give him or her a clearer idea of what you seek. A superior doctor will use this information to fine-tune your consultation in order to develop your customized breast augmentation plan.

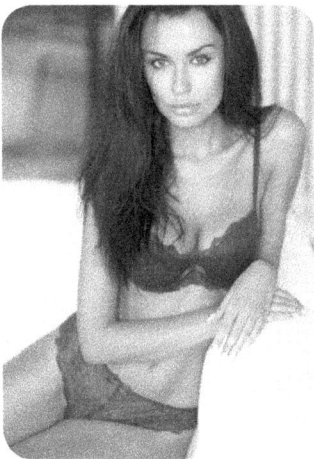

FIGURE 5.9 Lingerie tends to push breasts together and higher. This, in combination with the woman's pose and the position of her arms, accentuates her cleavage. (This is a model and not a patient.)

Narrowing Your Implant Search

Once you've clearly expressed to your surgeon the result you would like, both of you will discuss implant options. To review your options, read chapter 4. In this section we'll explore two common paths patients take: surgeon driven and patient driven.

Surgeon-Driven Approach

This is the "doctor knows best" strategy where patients hand over responsibility to the expert. In other words, they defer the choice of implant to their surgeon.

Left to her own devices, a patient may feel completely unqualified to pick the perfect implant out of a mind-numbing number of options—as you've learned earlier, there are over two thousand choices. The surgeon-driven method requires little patient participation in the decision-making process.

This approach, however, has a huge downside. By ceding decision-making to their doctors, patients are risking an outcome that doesn't match what they'd hoped for.

"But if I've clearly stated what I want, isn't it my surgeon's responsibility to make it happen?" you may ask.

The reality is many implants could look great, be proportional, and suit your body. Thus, a range of implants will look beautiful, not just one. As much as it would streamline your implant decision-making process, there is no such thing as one perfect implant size for you. To understand how a doctor can interpret a patient's desired outcome differently from the patient herself, we need to explore breast augmentation a bit deeper.

Let's say Jennifer's surgeon has determined all implants ranging from 300 to 400 cc would look great on her. The difference is the 300 cc implant may make her a full B cup, while the 400 cc implant may make her a full C cup, and the sizes in between would create a range of breast fullness between those two cup sizes. Following the surgeon-driven approach, Jennifer defers the decision to the doctor. As a result, he chooses an implant that makes Jennifer a full C cup. The procedure was successfully performed, and the result looks great. But when Jennifer sees her breasts, she's disappointed. "They look bigger than I really wanted them to be," she tells herself.

To avoid Jennifer's predicament, I recommend you take an active role in choosing your implant.

> Remember, this is your body!
> So it's your responsibility to make
> the decision that's best for you.

The bottom line is no matter how brilliant and famous a surgeon is, you're the only one who knows what result will satisfy you. This is why I recommend you avoid the surgeon-driven approach and embrace the patient-driven one instead.

Patient-Driven Approach

When you actively participate in choosing your implant, you're increasing the likelihood of experiencing a result you'll be thrilled with. In this section, you'll learn the pluses and minuses of various strategies to help you determine your implant size.

BAGS OF WATER OR RICE

Taking a practice run with an implant size can help you figure out the right size for you. One method is to fill plastic bags with water or rice. You'll find numerous Internet articles describing this technique. Many websites provide guidelines to determine how much water or rice you need to create a particular implant size in cubic centimeters.

The advantage of this approach is it's easy and practically free, and you can practice at home.

Unfortunately, in my experience working with patients, bags of water or rice are inaccurate assessment tools because the cc that patients select after experimenting with this approach often doesn't provide the look they seek.

One reason behind the discrepancy is the water or rice conversions may vary depending on the website you reference. As you know, the Internet is full of unscientific and unverified information. So while you may follow the water or rice measurement on the website, it may not be accurate in predicting which implant size you should choose. Basically, you're trusting that whoever published the information on the website is providing reliable information.

Another reason the water or rice approach is flawed is the way that the bags appear *outside* your body is dramatically different from how your breasts will appear when the implants are *inside* your body. Allow me to explain.

During surgery, most implants are placed below the muscle. The result is the implant will appear slightly smaller inside the breast in comparison to anything you practice wearing outside the breast. Websites and surgeons attempt to address the discrepancy between an implant below the muscle and a filled bag you practice with. For example, they'll say: *Subtract 30 cc from the final size you picked as a result of your practice run.*

But this is an inaccurate measurement because an implant has many variables influencing how it will look on your body. Thus it might be 20 cc, 30 cc, or 40 cc less than your bag of water or rice.

Similarly, filled bags appear quite differently compared to actual breast implants, which are advanced medical devices comprising special properties built into their shells. In the case of silicone implants, the silicone fill has characteristics that create its particular shape.

A simple bag of water or rice can never replicate this sophisticated technology.

So although the filled bags offer an inexpensive way to explore your size options, your efforts run the risk of providing you misleading information.

Next, the actual placement of your bags of water or rice poses another problem. Because they have to be held in place inside a bra, you can't see what your new breast size will look like when you're nude. Most of my patients identify this as a significant drawback—they want to see how their new breast size will appear without a bra.

Weight is another major flaw with bags of water or rice. When you pick up silicone or saline implants, you can feel their weight. But when they're actually inside the body, their weight is far less noticeable. In fact, after recovering, patients often tell me they can't feel the implant at all and even forget it's in their body. On the other hand, when women practice with bags of water or rice in a bra, the bags pull on the bra. The sensation is much heavier than that of an implant in the body.

Many of my patients became so concerned after feeling the weight of the bags they practiced with that they opted for smaller implants than they would have otherwise selected—even after I explained the flaws of the bags of water or rice approach *and* I recommended they not choose a smaller size. Unfortunately, after their breast augmentations many of these women wished they had followed my advice.

SIZING BRAS

For many years a sizing bra, which is designed to hold actual implants or a model of an implant, was the best way to help patients pick a size. In fact, this was the strategy I used with my patients when I first began my practice.

The advantage of sizing bras is they are more accurate than the water or rice technique. They'll give you a reasonable idea of what you'll look like with any given implant size.

But sizing bras have the following drawbacks, which are similar to those of bags of water or rice:

- The way the implants appear *outside* your body is dramatically different from how your breasts will appear when the implants are *inside* your body.

- During your practice run, the implants are held inside a sizing bra, so you can't see what your new breast size will look like without a bra.

- When you practice with implants in a sizing bra, the implants pull on the bra. The sensation is much heavier than that of an implant in the body.

In summary, sizing bras are a mediocre way to choose an implant. Using them causes many women to choose implants much smaller than they really would have otherwise selected.

3D IMAGING

In the past, I've suggested my patients try both approaches: bags of water or rice and sizing bras. While these methods had their drawbacks, they were the best options available at the time. But thanks to cutting-edge technology, a new approach is available. Three-dimensional imaging has dramatically improved the ability to accurately select an implant size.

What Is 3D Imaging and How Does It Work?

This advanced technology provides a digital simulation of your breast augmentation results. Three-dimensional imaging uses high-resolution cameras, which take detailed photos of a patient's breasts from various angles. Within seconds, sophisticated computer software processes the photos to create a three-dimensional image of your breasts (see figures 5.10 and 5.11).

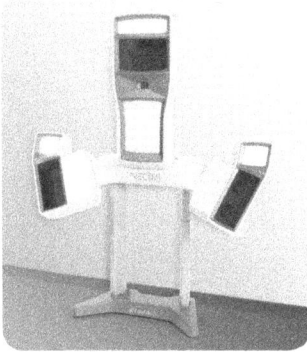

FIGURE 5.10. The Vectra 3D imaging system.

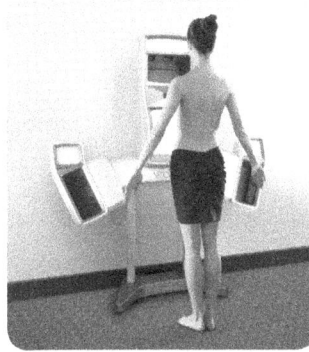

FIGURE 5.11. The patient stands in front of the camera system, and a series of images are taken. The images are then processed to create a 3D image of the patient.

You can then see 3D images of all implant options available including saline, silicone, round, anatomic, smooth, and textured implants.

With 3D imaging, you're able to view what a particular implant will look like on your body from multiple angles. From there, you can perform side-by-side comparisons of the implant options you're considering (see figures 5.12 and 5.13).

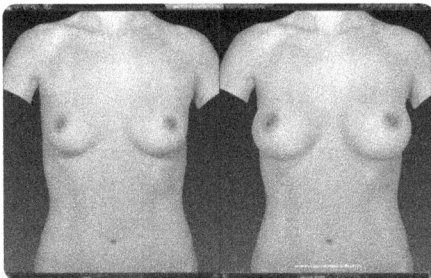

FIGURE 5.12. An example of a 3D simulation created by the Vectra. The picture on the right shows the patient what she will look like with the selected implant size.

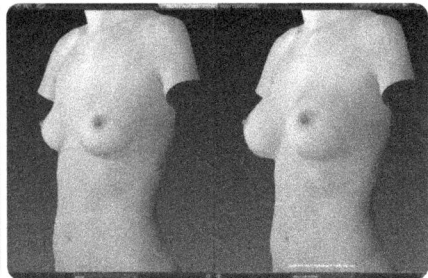

FIGURE 5.13. Another view of the same patient.

3D Imaging Advantages

Compared to the patient feedback I've received and the surgical results I've experienced after having thousands of patients practice using filled bags and sizing bras, I can confidently say the benefits of 3D imaging are unmatched. No other approach has worked better or satisfied my patients more.

The main reason I believe 3D imaging is superior is it allows you to see how an implant will look on your body when you're not wearing clothes or a bra. In contrast, other methods require a bra or clothing to hold a bag of water or rice or an implant in place. So none of these approaches provide an accurate image of what you'll look like nude.

Also, 3D imaging allows the surgeon to achieve the best **symmetry** possible. Symmetry refers to the degree to which your two breasts will look the same. Every woman has slight differences between her two breasts and the two sides of her chest. For example, one breast may be slightly bigger than the other breast. Because 3D imaging provides detailed measurements of the breast size and position, the surgeon has the information necessary to plan ahead and make adjustments to the size of the implants and their positioning. The result is breasts that are as symmetric as possible.

The 3D imaging also simulates other essential details about your result. For example, most women who seek breast augmentation are concerned about the amount of space (also called cleavage) they will have between their breasts. The benefit of 3D imaging is it generates a realistic image of your breasts and the amount of cleavage you can expect.

With 3D imaging, you're able to see what your breasts will look like when you're nude, it provides the surgeon with precise measurements for a better result, and it shows you the most realistic and accurate simulation possible of what you can expect after surgery.

Will the Implant Fit?

A final step in choosing an implant size is making sure it will actually fit inside the breast. As you've learned earlier, implants come in a wide variety of shapes. Each shape has specific measurements associated with it. One of the most important measurements of a breast implant is its **base width.**

The implant's base width is the width, or diameter, of the part of the implant that's in contact with your chest. This measurement is extremely important because it must be equal to, or less than, the width of each of your breasts. In other words, the width of the implant should match the width of the breast.

If the implant width is equal to your breast width, or if it's smaller, then it will most likely fit comfortably inside the breast allowing your breast tissues to drape around it beautifully. If, however, the width of the implant is wider than the width of the breast, then it will most likely not fit comfortably inside the breast and the breast tissues will not drape nicely. This increases the chances of irregularities, complications, and disappointing results. For example, an implant that is too wide for the breast has to essentially be stuffed inside the breast to fit. This can create an unnatural bulge on the side or the bottom of the breast.

Another important measurement is the implant's **projection**; this refers to how far the implant sticks out (or projects) from the chest. The bigger the implant projection, the more it stretches the breast skin.

For the low profile, moderate-plus profile, and gummy bear implants, skin stretching is typically not a significant issue because these implants have less projection than other implants (for more on implant profiles refer to chapter 4). Skin stretching plays a bigger role in high profile and extra-high profile implants because they are rounder and have more projection compared to other implants of the same width.

Every woman's breast skin has a limit to how much it can be stretched. Some women have breast skin that can be easily stretched, while other women have tighter breast skin that can't be stretched very much. During the consultation, your surgeon should measure how much breast-skin stretch you have. This will ensure your breasts can handle the amount of projection the implant has.

Thus, the last step in choosing an implant is to make sure its measurements match the measurements of your breast. Confirming that the width and projection of the implant are appropriate for the width and skin stretch of your breast will ensure you will experience a beautiful result.

Summary

- The final size you will be after breast augmentation depends on various factors. These include your height, weight, the amount of breast tissue you begin with, the shape of your breasts before surgery, and the size and shape of the implant selected.

- There is no such thing as a perfect size. Each woman has a range of sizes that will all create a beautiful result.

- Cup sizes can't be guaranteed. You may be a C cup for one brand of bra, a full C for another brand, and a small D for yet another brand. Cup sizes can even vary within the same brand, depending on the style.

- I recommend the patient-driven approach to choosing an implant. This method actively involves you in the implant selection process. As a result, you'll increase the chances you will love your outcome.

- Three-dimensional imaging is the most reliable and successful way to select an implant size.

- The dimensions of the implant must match your breast width and breast-skin stretching ability.

To find the implant size that will give you the look you dream of requires a thorough consultation with a surgeon who can explain your multiple options using 3D imaging. By following the recommendations in this chapter, you're on your way to selecting the implant size that will provide you with a beautiful result for years to come.

In the next chapter, I will review how implants are placed within the breast and the advantages and disadvantages of each option.

Breast Augmentation Myths

My cup size will be guaranteed after my breast augmentation.

Unfortunately, there is no way to guarantee a specific bra size. The main reason is bra cup sizes vary tremendously depending on which brand of bra you buy. For instance, you can be a C cup in one brand and a D cup in another brand. You can even be different cup sizes within the same brand depending on which style of bra you buy.

The best any surgeon can do is provide you an estimate of the cup size you should be for most bra companies. For example, a surgeon can estimate you should be around a C cup with a certain size implant for most bra companies. But keep in mind this means you may be a small C, average C, full C, or even a small D, depending on the bra brand you buy.

This is why it's important your surgeon offers 3D imaging, which will simulate your result when you're nude. If you're happy with the way you look in the simulation, then you increase the likelihood you'll be happy with the surgical outcome, no matter what bra you buy.

There is one perfect size implant for me.

The truth is many implant styles and shapes have the potential to look great on you. So, rather than just one, several sizes will provide a beautiful result.

The goal of surgery is to provide you with a look that will make you happy. The tricky part is what makes one patient happy can be dramatically different from what makes another patient happy. Thus, using a one-size-fits-all approach to breast augmentation doesn't work. In other words, you can't apply the same strategy to every individual. Each patient needs a custom surgical plan.

This is why a thorough consultation is so important. Describing your goals to the surgeon and providing pictures of the results that appeal to you are critical to achieving a great result.

Once the surgeon understands what your goals are, he or she can make specific recommendations designed for you. A surgeon's expertise combined with 3D imaging will help you understand what you can expect with each implant choice.

In the end, the perfect implant size is one that will give you the result *YOU* want. A top surgeon will work closely with you. He or she will carefully listen to and understand what your goals are. Together, through clear communication, patient education, thorough exams, and 3D imaging, you'll develop a plan to make your breast augmentation dreams come true.

CHAPTER 6

IMPLANT PLACEMENT

In this chapter, you'll learn:

- essential aspects of your anatomy that are relevant to your implant placement decision;

- your implant placement options;

- the advantages and disadvantages of implant placement options.

Real Conversations

Six months after Rachel had undergone breast augmentation with another surgeon, she made an appointment to see me. She was dissatisfied with her surgical result and wanted a second opinion.

"After my body healed, I was happy with Dr. Smith's work," she told me. "But now, I'm convinced my left breast is firmer than my right. During my follow-up appointment, I told Dr. Smith about this, and he reassured me everything was fine. But I don't think every-thing is fine, so I wanted you to take a look."

"Do you know if your implants are over or under the muscle?" I asked.

"I'm not sure. Should I know this?" she asked.

"It's certainly something you and your doctor should have talked about," I said.

Rachel didn't recall any conversation about this. I then briefly examined her breasts and concluded her implants were over the muscle. I explained that the firmness she was experiencing was most likely capsular contracture, which is the hardening of the scar around the implant. This commonly occurs when implants are placed over the muscle.

"Oh no!" Rachel said. "I would have *never* agreed to have implants over the muscle if I knew this could happen. I wish the other doctor had explained this to me."

Introduction

In my practice, I regularly see patients who are in a predicament similar to Rachel's. They are unhappy with the result of their breast augmentation surgery they underwent with another doctor, and they're seeking a second opinion. In some cases, the problem is a poorly performed procedure. But in most instances, the patient's dissatisfaction is the consequence of insufficient communication. For example, a patient and her surgeon may have never had an over-the-muscle versus under-the-muscle conversation. To avoid encountering problems that result from poor communication, in this chapter, you'll learn about the various implant placement options and their advantages and disadvantages.

Chest Anatomy Made Simple

Once you've chosen an implant, you must next decide whether the implant should be placed over or under the muscle. In order to understand the advantages and disadvantages of each, you need a basic background of the chest and breast anatomy. Rather than complicated and unnecessarily technical explanations, this section will provide straightforward information regarding your body.

FOUR LAYERS OF YOUR CHEST

Imagine you had superhero X-ray vision and were looking at your body in a mirror. Using your superpowers, you'd see skin, muscles, and bones. If you looked directly at your breasts, you'd see four layers:

1. The superficial skin, including the skin of the nipple and areola.

2. Subcutaneous tissue, which is the thin layer of fat tissue beneath the skin. This layer also contains the breast gland.

3. Muscle.

4. Ribcage.

Please refer to figure 6.1 to see how these layers look.

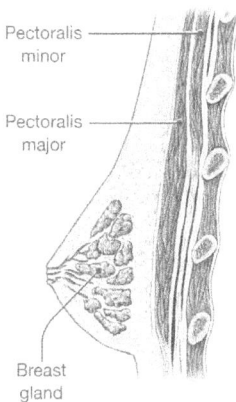

FIGURE 6.1.
Basic anatomy of the breast.

Pectoralis minor

Pectoralis major

Breast gland

The first layer is the **superficial skin,** including the nipple and areola. At a thickness of less than one centimeter, it is very thin.

The second layer is the **subcutaneous tissue.** "Sub" means below, and "cutaneous" means skin. This is the layer directly below the skin. The subcutaneous tissue comprises fat cells. The thickness of this layer varies greatly from person to person. In general, the heavier a woman is, the more fat cells that are beneath the skin. And the thinner the woman is, the fewer fat cells that are beneath the skin.

The breast gland is located within the subcutaneous layer. The breast gland is distributed around the entire female breast. This is the tissue that produces milk in response to hormones released during pregnancy.

Within the breast are millions of tiny milk ducts, nerves, and blood vessels—all of which run in multiple directions and are part of the breast tissue. Most of these milk ducts, nerves, and blood vessels are invisible to the naked eye.

The third layer is the **muscle.** Throughout our bodies, we have many muscle groups. The chest muscle is called the pectoralis muscle. It is the main chest muscle and one that allows you to do push-ups or any other action that involves pushing straight out with your arms or bringing your arms together to the center of your chest.

The pectoralis muscle is strong and varies in thickness. If you regularly perform chest exercises, it can be thick. If you don't exercise your chest muscles much, it can be very thin. But even the thinnest pectoralis muscle is still about a quarter of an inch thick.

The fourth layer is the bones of the **ribcage.** The ribcage provides a strong protective layer around the organs of the chest.

Implant Placement

- Over the muscle (subglandular)

- Under the muscle (submuscular)

- Dual plane

- Subfascial

As you've learned, the four breast layers are the superficial skin (including the skin of the nipple and areola), the subcutaneous tissue, muscle, and ribcage. An over-the-muscle implant will be below the breast gland tissue and above the muscle. For this reason, it is commonly referred to as the subglandular position—"sub" means below, and "glandular" refers to the breast gland. So when you hear "subglandular position," it is the same as "over the muscle."

Before and after implants: profile view

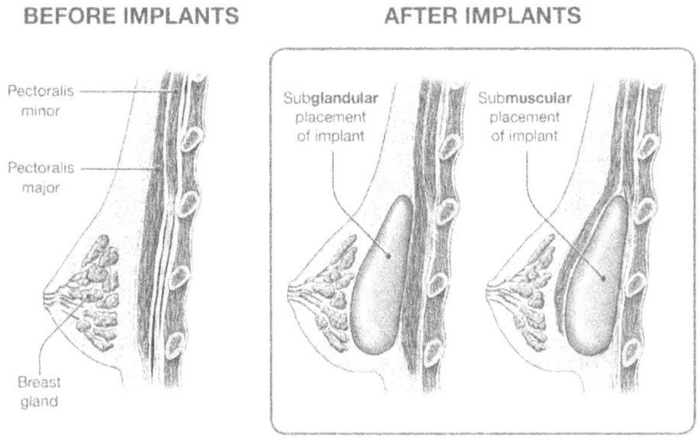

BEFORE IMPLANTS   AFTER IMPLANTS

Pectoralis minor

Pectoralis major

Subglandular placement of implant

Submuscular placement of implant

Breast gland

FIGURE 6.2. A side view of subglandular and submuscular placement of implants.

In contrast, when an implant is placed *below* the muscle, it is called "submuscular." (See figures 6.2 and 6.3.) So when you hear "submuscular position," it is the same as "below the muscle." The dual plane and subfascial plane positions will be explained later in this chapter.

Placement of implants: front view

SUBGLANDULAR   SUBMUSCULAR

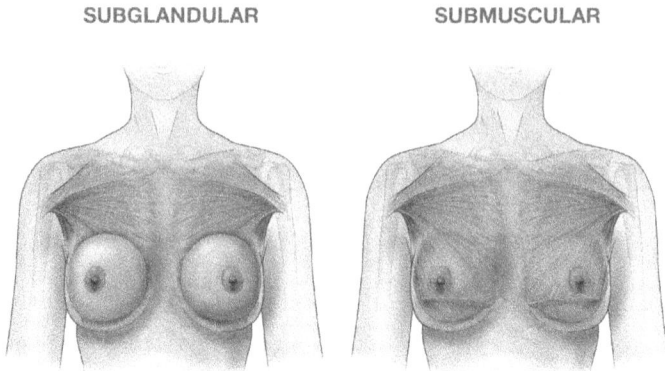

FIGURE 6.3. A front view of subglandular and submuscular placement of implants.

SUBGLANDULAR POSITION

Overview

More than forty years ago, when breast augmentation surgery began, most surgeons placed implants in the subglandular (over-the-muscle) position. It seemed the most logical location because, from a surgical perspective, creating a space between the muscle and the breast gland was a relatively simple procedure to perform.

This is because the muscle and the breast gland are attached to each other by very thin fibers. The surgeon can easily open these fibers to create a space for the implant. Once the surgeon creates the space, he or she places an implant in the opening. The fibers around the pocket of space are left intact, and they're strong enough to keep the breast gland attached to the muscle and the implant in its place.

Advantages

As you learned, separating the thin fibers holding the breast gland from the muscle layer below is a relatively straightforward surgical procedure. Thus, placing the implant over the muscle is generally a quick and easy technique to perform.

Another advantage of a subglandular procedure is the postoperative recovery may be slightly easier compared to a submuscular procedure. This is because submuscular placement requires manipulating the muscle tissue, which may result in slightly more pain after your surgery. But overall, the recovery time difference between the two is minimal.

Next, the subglandular position is better for women who are professional body builders. The reason is submuscular-implant placement requires cutting part of the muscle fibers to make space for the implant. If women who lift heavy weights opt for a submuscular procedure, they may notice a decrease in strength afterwards. Therefore, they may not be able to lift the same amount of weight they did before the surgery. Thus, for this small and specific group of individuals, the subglandular placement may be best.

With that said, for the vast majority of women, the submuscular procedure does not affect their strength or ability to exercise. For example, many patients in my Beverly Hills practice are highly fit and have a regular exercise routine. None of them who have undergone a submuscular procedure has difficulty returning to her usual workout after she has recovered from surgery.

Disadvantages

Compared to patients who undergo submuscular procedures, women with subglandular implants experience a higher rate of complications over time. First, when implants are placed above the muscle, the implant's edges often become visible and noticeable. This happens because the only tissue covering an implant is the skin and breast gland, and most women undergoing breast augmentation have a small amount of breast tissue to begin with. The very fact that they have a small amount of breast tissue is why they are seeking breast augmentation in the first place. When women can see and feel an implant's edges, they usually express concern and disappointment with their breast augmentation result.

Second, subglandular implants also frequently result in visible rippling. Again, this happens because a subglandular implant has very little tissue covering it. So over time, even if the rippling is minor, most women will feel and see it on their skin's surface.

Another complication with subglandular implants is an increased risk of hardening and distortion of the breasts. This is called capsular contracture (see figure 6.4). Studies have shown the rate of capsular contracture is much higher when implants are placed *over* the muscle compared to implants placed *below* the muscle.

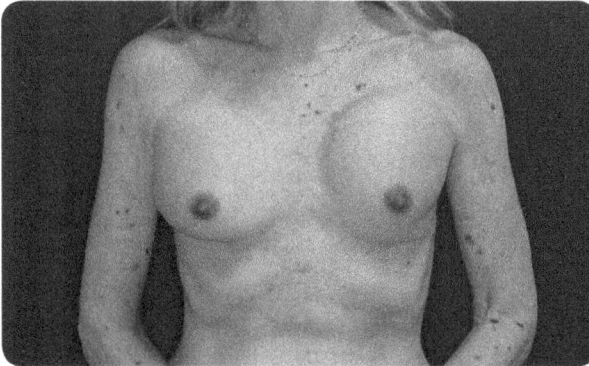

FIGURE 6.4. An example of a patient with capsular contracture of the breasts.

SUBMUSCULAR POSITION
Overview

Submuscular placement means that the implant is placed within a pocket under the muscle of the chest. (Review figures 6.2 and 6.3.)

In order to place an implant under the muscle, the muscle fibers at the bottom of the chest must be opened. This allows the surgeon to lift the muscle and create an open space for the implant. Once the implant is inserted, it is located below the muscle and above the ribcage.

Advantages

As a result of the numerous problems associated with implants placed above the muscle, surgeons began placing implants under the muscle. This approach offered several advantages.

When the implant is placed below the muscle, the implant has an additional layer of cushion above it. This layer of muscle prevents the implant's edges from becoming visible over time. As a result, the likelihood of visible edges and rippling are much lower than with implants placed in the subglandular position.

The most important advantage of submuscular implants, however, is that it prevents capsular contracture. Although the reason why is not fully understood, women with implants in the submuscular position are much less likely to develop hardening and distortion of their breasts. With that said, placing implants in the submuscular space does not guarantee that capsular contracture will never happen. It does, however, have a significantly lower likelihood that you'll experience it.

Disadvantages

One possible drawback of submuscular placement is **animation displacement**. This refers to the visible movement of the implant when the chest muscle contracts (see figure 6.5).

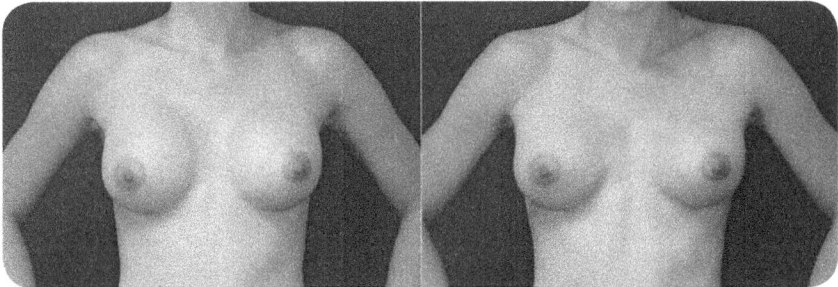

FIGURE 6.5. An example of animation displacement. The patient is contracting her pectoralis muscle on the right side of the image. When this happens, the muscle pushes on the implants and makes the implants move slightly outward.

When an implant is placed under the muscle and the muscle presses on it, the implant tends to move downward and outward. Although this is a common occurrence, it is considered a minor side effect and rarely, if ever, causes any problems. Nevertheless, a thorough assessment of your options means you should be aware of it.

DUAL PLANE

When you look at the picture of a breast implant in the submuscular space, pay particular attention to the following points. First, notice that the muscle's bottom edge runs at a diagonal below the level of the nipple (see figure 6.6). This is because during surgery, the muscle has been opened to allow space for an implant to fit. As a result, no pectoralis muscle is present in the area at the bottom of the breast. Second, the implant has to be positioned so it's centered behind the nipple. This is to ensure that the breast has a natural shape.

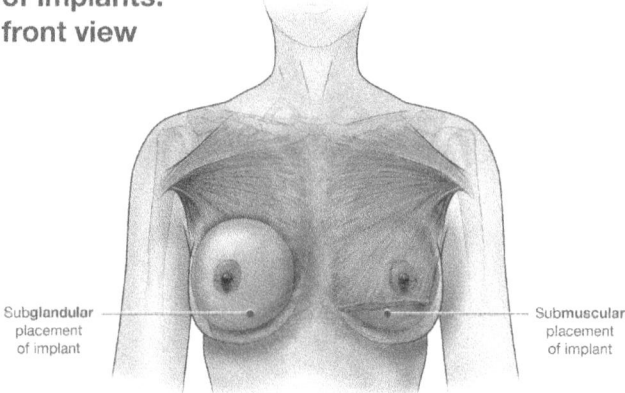

Placement of implants: front view

Subglandular placement of implant

Submuscular placement of implant

FIGURE 6.6. Front view of subglandular and submuscular implant placement. Notice that in a submuscular placement (shown on the right) the upper two-thirds of the implant is covered by muscle but the bottom third of the implant is not covered by muscle. The bottom third is covered by breast tissue and skin only. This is described as a "dual plane" because the implant is under two (dual) different tissues.

When you combine the first and second points, the upper two-thirds of the implant will be above the level of the nipple, and the lower third of the implant will be below the level of the nipple. Please refer to figure 6.6 again to review the anatomy.

As you can see in the diagram, muscle covers the upper two thirds of the implant, but it doesn't cover the lower one third of the implant. In other words, muscle covers the upper part of the implant, and breast tissue covers the lower part of the implant. Because two different tissues cover the implant, this placement is referred to as a dual plane.

A dual plane occurs anytime the implant is placed in the sub-muscular (below-the-muscle) position. Thus, any under-the-muscle implant is automatically in the dual plane. So when you read or hear about a dual plane implant, it means the same as the implant being in the submuscular (under-the-muscle) position.

Surgeons have created different categories for dual plane procedures that appear in a grading system: dual plane one, two, and three. The difference between dual plane one, two, and three is beyond the scope of this book. Just remember all implants placed under the muscle are automatically placed in a dual plane.

SUBFASCIAL PLANE

"Fascial" refers to **fascia,** which is an extremely thin sheet of tissue that covers the pectoralis muscle. Fascia actually covers all your body's muscles. Some surgeons advertise they can place the implant in the layer above the muscle and below its fascia, hence the "sub" in "subfascial." They often claim this approach provides patients all the benefits of an under-the-muscle procedure without opening the muscle.

A subfascial plane breast augmentation is a difficult, if not impossible, procedure to execute successfully because the fascia is an extremely thin tissue. Dissecting it requires an extraordinary level of precision and time. It would be like trying to peel a grape's skin without ever tearing it. Even the most experienced and skilled plastic surgeons will inadvertently tear the fascia when they attempt to separate it from the muscle. What's worse, tearing often creates little holes that bleed.

A subfascial plane procedure is typically only used in complicated breast revision surgery because these women may not have normal and healthy muscle tissue for coverage of the implant.

Even if a surgeon assures you he or she is experienced at performing subfascial plane operations, your fascia is highly likely to tear in multiple places before the implant is inserted. As a result, a flimsy and damaged fascia will likely cover an implant placed in a subfascial plane. In this case, you'll experience none of the benefits of having an implant placed under the muscle and all of the risks associated with a poorly performed procedure.

Summary

- Implants can be placed within a pocket over the muscle or under the muscle.

- Subglandular implants are located between the breast gland and the pectoralis muscle.

- Submuscular implants are located between the muscle and the rib cage.

- The advantages of placing an implant under the muscle (submuscular) have made this approach the standard practice in today's breast augmentations.

- Subglandular placement of implants increases the risk of complications, such as rippling and capsular contracture.

- The dual plane position and the submuscular position are essentially the same.

- A subfascial position is very difficult to achieve. It is mainly used for complicated breast revision or breast reconstruction cases. It is unnecessary for cosmetic breast augmentation.

Excellent board-certified plastic surgeons will explain your placement options to you. They will describe the advantages and advantages of different approaches. If your prospective doctor fails to provide you essential guidance, look elsewhere.

In the next chapter, you will learn the options you have regarding where implants are inserted, the advantages and disadvantages of each insertion point, and the importance of scar design.

Breast Augmentation Myths

Placing the implant over the muscle will give me a breast lift.

Patients who have looseness of their breast skin as a result of weight loss or breastfeeding or both often come into my office having heard this myth. They believe that by placing their implants over the muscle, the so-called lifting aspect of this procedure will make a separate breast lift surgery unnecessary.

Nothing could be further from the truth.

While implants placed over the muscle may initially make the breasts appear perkier, this is because the implant temporarily stretches out the loose skin. Implants placed under the muscle also temporarily stretch out the skin, although to a slightly lesser extent.

In both instances—over and under the muscle—any perceived perkiness is temporary. Once the swelling from the procedure decreases, the breast skin will begin to relax and become loose again. Over time, the entire breast, implant and all, will drop to a lower position. Put simply, a subglandular implant will not create any long-lasting lifting of the breast.

If a woman needs a breast lift, does not have one done, and undergoes a subglandular breast augmentation, the breast's appearance will be worse than it was prior to surgery for two reasons: First, because the implant does not have the benefit of a muscle covering it, the implant's edges will be visible. Thus, the weight of the implant will pull the breast down, and the outline of the implant will become noticeable. Second, without a breast lift, the breast's shape hasn't been improved. Either way, the result will be unattractive and unsatisfactory.

If you have loose skin as a result of weight loss or breastfeeding or both, you'll most likely need a breast lift in addition to the augmentation—regardless of whether the placement is over or under the muscle. Simply placing the implant over the muscle in hopes of inflating the breast skin will not work. Any improvement you'll see afterwards will be only temporary.

Placing the implant over the muscle is safer and easier compared to placing it under the muscle.

Although placing an implant over the muscle (also called the "subglandular position") simplifies the procedure for the surgeon, it is not safer for the patient over the long run. Implants placed over the muscle expose you to an increased likelihood of visible edges, rippling, and capsular contracture, which is the hardening of the scar around the implant.

A top board certified plastic surgeon who performs a high number of breast augmentations will easily and safely insert the implant under the muscle. Doing so will be his or her preference because the long-term benefits far outweigh the risks associated with a subglandu-lar implant placement. The bottom line is having a submuscular implant will provide you with a more beautiful and safer long-lasting result.

CHAPTER 7

INCISION LOCATION

In this chapter, you'll learn:

- what the various options are for the location of the incision;

- the advantages and disadvantages of each option;

- common myths and misconceptions about incisions and scars.

Real Conversations

After researching extensively about breast augmentation, Hannah was sure she wanted to undergo the procedure. She found a surgeon who advertised a "scarless technique." The thought of having no scar appealed to her, so she scheduled a consultation right away.

During Hannah's appointment, Dr. Stuart explained that his special approach involved inserting implants through the bellybutton.

Dr. Stuart highlighted the technique's multiple benefits, which motivated Hannah to schedule her surgery on the spot.

When Hannah arrived home that day, she searched online to learn more about the scarless procedure. As she had done previously when researching breast augmentation, she visited the American Society of Plastic Surgeons (ASPS) website. Unfortunately, she couldn't find any information about it there.

She then searched other sites. Hannah learned the bellybutton approach had a high complication rate and the ASPS didn't recognize it as a safe procedure—this explained why it didn't appear on the ASPS site.

Hannah was both disappointed and relieved with her discovery: While she wished Dr. Stuart's strategy was a safe option, she was glad she had found out about the significant risks associated with the belly-button procedure before she had the surgery. Hannah immediately cancelled her surgery appointment.

Introduction

"Dr. Diaz, will I have a scar?" patients frequently ask me. In fact, scarring is one of the biggest concerns women have in regards to their breast augmentation. Patients want to know where and how big their scar will be and what it will look like.

Their worries make sense. After all, most of us want to avoid scarring as much as possible. We often associate scars with accidents and surgeries we had to undergo in order to stay healthy. In these instances, scarring was largely out of our control. But in breast augmentation, a scar is an integral part of the procedure itself.

All high quality breast augmentation surgeons emphasize scar placement and design—yes, the scar is intentionally planned. While this design element may sound off-putting because what you probably seek is no scar at all, such a perspective is unrealistic. If a surgeon could perform a breast augmentation without a scar, then he or she would be a magician. And if a doctor promises a scarless outcome, you should run the other way!

In recent years, many brilliant surgeons have advanced breast augmentations to new heights. They have devised innovative and creative ways to leave little scarring. While all board-certified plastic surgeons have learned how to design incisions, the best plastic surgeons pride themselves on their ability to minimize a scar's appearance, and they have a long track record to demonstrate the superiority of their technique.

In this chapter, you'll learn about the different options you have when it comes to deciding where to insert an implant. We'll explore the advantages and disadvantages of each, including the design and placement of scars.

Overview: Four Implant Insertion Points

In this section, I'll refer to **submuscular** and **subglandular implant placement**, which you learned about earlier. Please read chapter 6 to review these important terms. Next, keep in mind the following as you read this section:

> The longer the distance between the breast tissue and the implant insertion point, the more complicated the procedure becomes and the greater number of risks you'll encounter.

Also, when it comes to breast implant insertion, three factors are essential to creating a beautiful breast augmentation result:

1. The amount of visibility a surgeon has of the space where the implant is placed

2. The degree to which the surgeon can control the shape of the pocket within the breast tissue where the implant is placed

3. The fact that the breast's shape will be largely controlled by the degree to which the surgeon can control the shape of the pocket

Breast implants are inserted in one of the following four points (see figure 7.1):

- Bellybutton (or umbilicus)

- Armpit (or axilla)

- Nipple (or areola)

- Breast crease (also called an inframammary crease or inframammary fold) at the bottom of the breast

Incisions: front view

FIGURE 7.1. Incision options for breast implant insertion.

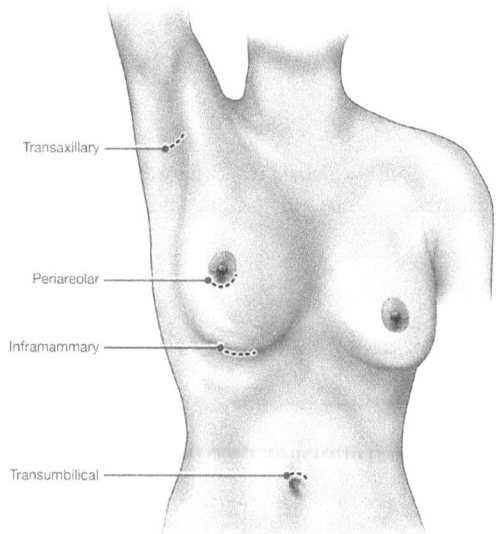

Transaxillary

Periareolar

Inframammary

Transumbilical

The incisions for all insertion points measure about 1.25 inches. Accommodating the size of the surgical instruments is the reason behind this length.

BELLYBUTTON (OR UMBILICUS)

The technical name for inserting implants through the bellybutton is called "trans-umbilical breast augmentation," or TUBA. "Trans" means through, and "umbilical" refers to the bellybutton. This procedure first appeared in the plastic surgery literature twenty years ago.

In TUBA, the scar remains largely hidden because it curves along the inner part of the bellybutton. Bellybutton scars also tend to heal well. And on the breast itself, no scars are actually created.

As with all breast augmentation techniques, there are two options for implant placement. One is above the muscle. This position is called subglandular. The second is below the muscle. This position is called submuscular.

TUBA procedures require inserting an outer tube into the body that begins at the bellybutton and extends to the breast tissue. Once the outer tube is set in place, it acts as a tunnel for a smaller instrument that travels through it (see figure 7.2).

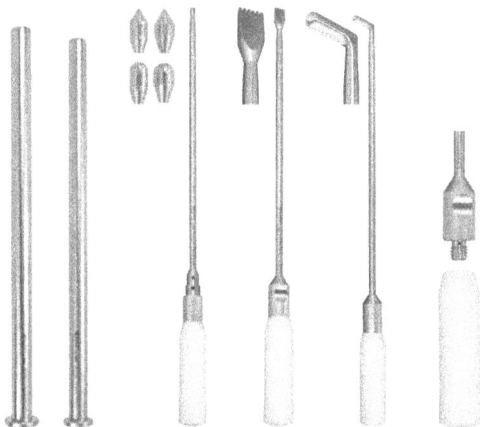

FIGURE 7.2. Instruments used in a TUBA procedure. (Permission granted by Integra LifeSciences Corporation, Plainsboro, New Jersey, USA.)

Subglandular TUBA

The surgeon starts by making a bellybutton incision that serves as the entry point for a hollow tube-shaped instrument. This is placed in between the abdominal muscle and the abdominal skin. From there, it's pushed to the breast tissue. Pushing the tube into the subglandular position from the bellybutton to the breast is relatively easy because the tube travels along the same layer of tissue from beginning to end.

Submuscular TUBA

As you read in a previous chapter, placing implants under the muscle is the ideal position. But in a TUBA, doing so adds a significant layer of complexity and risk to your procedure. This is because the surgeon has to manipulate the tube from one layer to another. Once the tube is advanced from the bellybutton to the breast, it is by default in the subglandular position. However, if the implant will be placed in the submuscular position, the surgeon must change the position of the tube. To do so, the surgeon typically pierces the chest muscle using the tube itself. The surgeon must do this blindly because he or she has no way of seeing the chest muscle from the tube's bellybutton insertion point. Because this procedure requires many complicated steps, there are significant risks associated with this approach.

Outer Tube and Instrument

The main outer tube serves as a tunnel for a smaller instrument that travels inside it. The smaller instrument has a long handle and a tip with flat ends. Once the smaller instrument has reached the breast, the surgeon gently moves the instrument from side to side to create a pocket inside the breast. If the tube is in the subglandular position, the newly formed pocket will be in the subglandular position. If the tube is in the submuscular position, the newly formed pocket will be in the submuscular position.

The surgeon then removes the smaller instrument and prepares to insert the saline implants. Only saline implants can be used in the TUBA because saline implants are empty at first. In this deflated state, they are small enough to travel inside the outer tube to the breast. In contrast, because silicone implants are already filled, they are too big to travel inside the outer tube.

The surgeon rolls the saline shell into a cigar-like shape, which will be able to fit inside the outer tube and travel through it. The saline implants themselves have a long, thin, flexible filling tube temporarily attached to them. This tube looks like a drinking straw and is used to fill the implant with saline.

A small instrument is used to push the saline implant through the inside of the outer tube. After the implant reaches the proper position within the breast, the surgeon then fills the implant with saline, the filling tube is removed, the implant's opening is sealed, and the bellybutton incision is closed.

Multiple risks are associated with TUBA. First, because the distance between the bellybutton and the breast is long, many mishaps can occur when pushing multiple instruments and implants along the path. In rare instances, the instruments have pierced the abdomen or chest or both and have injured internal organs in the process.

Second, compared to other techniques, creating a subglandular or submuscular pocket for the implant's final position from an insertion point that starts at the bellybutton adds a layer of complexity to a breast augmentation. Remember, the surgeon must make sure the tube enters the correct breast layer. This is made difficult because he or she is unable to see precisely where the instruments are as they travel from the bellybutton to the breast tissue. In fact, the tube may actually travel up a different path than the doctor intended.

To my shock, I've seen patients who have undergone TUBA procedures where their surgeon accidentally placed an implant in the subglandular space on one side and in the submuscular space on the other side. These patients have come to me seeking a revision breast augmentation surgery. While they were not satisfied with their original surgeon's work, they had no idea of the true cause—that their doctor had made such an appalling mistake.

Even if the surgeon places the implants in the position he or she intended, the TUBA makes it difficult for the surgeon to control the pocket's shape where the implant will be placed. As a result, the surgeon is often unable to fine-tune the breast's shape once the implant is in its final position. This drawback can result in greater irregular breast contours or asymmetry or both compared to other approaches.

In a TUBA, the surgeon also has difficulty controlling or preventing bleeding. And excess bleeding during breast augmentation has been linked to increased risks for capsular contracture, which is the hardening and distortion of the breasts. This means the risk of capsular contracture may be higher with a TUBA procedure compared to other breast augmentation techniques.

Because of the multiple weaknesses of TUBAs, few surgeons perform them. In fact, the American Society of Plastic Surgeons does not recommend a TUBA. But despite the complications of this method, many surgeons still advertise their ability to perform these so-called scarless breast augmentations. But without exception, I advise my patients against inserting implants through the bellybutton.

Summary
A TUBA is one option for you. The benefit of minimal scarring and no scarring on the breast itself are this procedure's most appealing features. But experiencing the benefits of no scarring comes at significant risk. Although some patients can achieve a beautiful result, I've seen too many women come into my office with serious complications that arose from a TUBA.

ARMPIT (OR AXILLA)

Inserting implants through the armpit is called transaxillary breast augmentation. This approach is similar to a TUBA procedure in the following ways:

1. The incision is located relatively far from the breast.

2. Blunt tubes are used as instruments to create the breast pocket.

3. The surgeon does not have a direct view of all areas of the breast pocket being created.

Once the surgeon makes the incision in the armpit, he or she uses long tube-shaped instruments to form a pocket in the breast's subglandular or submuscular plane. The surgeon then inserts the implant and closes the incision.

Compared to the TUBA technique, the surgeon is better able to see where the instruments are as they travel from the armpit to the breast tissue. This is because the distance between the armpit and the breast is shorter than from the bellybutton to the breast.

Nevertheless, seeing the instrument's location is still awkward. For example, it is nearly impossible to view the outer side of the breast pocket from the armpit. This makes it difficult for the doctor to control the pocket's shape, which also makes it a challenge to control the breast's shape once the implant is in its final position. As a result, most doctors end up shaping this area by feel only—not the most precise strategy. This can result in irregular breast contours or asymmetry or both.

To overcome this weakness, some surgeons insert a small camera to see the breast pocket better. Unfortunately, using a camera is cumbersome, is time-consuming, and adds a layer of unnecessary complexity to a breast augmentation.

Furthermore, based on my experience, the scar is not signifi-cantly smaller or less visible than the scars made in the nipple or breast crease. Lastly, keep in mind the armpit skin has many sweat glands and follicles. These may contribute to the darkening of the scar. As a result, many patients wind up with dark scars that can be noticeable anytime they wear clothing, such as tank tops and strap-less dresses, that reveals their underarm area (see figure 7.3).

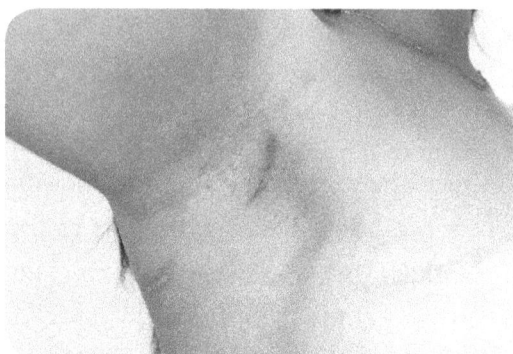

FIGURE 7.3. An axillary breast augmentation scar.

In summary, although the axillary approach is relatively safe, it still has many of the same disadvantages associated with a TUBA, such as increased risks of irregularities or asymmetry. Also, the scar can be dark and visible when you're wearing clothes that expose your underarm area.

NIPPLE (OR AREOLA)

For years, making a 1.25-inch incision along the edge of the bottom half of the areola (where the dark color of the area meets the light color of the breast) was the most common and sought-after breast augmentation technique.

After making the initial incision, the surgeon dissects the breast tissue to reach the muscle level. From there, the surgeon creates either a subglandular or submuscular pocket. The implant is then passed through the incision made along the areola and placed within the pocket. The incisions are then closed.

Compared to the bellybutton and armpit techniques, the areolar approach is considered safer. It also provides reliable and consistent results. The surgeon has high visibility of the entire breast pocket and can control the breast shape easily. The scar, although visible, is camouflaged by the color change between the darker areola and the lighter breast skin.

The main disadvantage of the areolar technique is it has been shown to have a high risk of capsular contracture. Although the causes of capsular contracture aren't fully known, one theory relates to bacterial infection. The areola and nipple have an irregular surface that is covered with tiny openings that lead into the milk ducts. Many of these openings can contain bacterial cells even after the skin's surface is carefully and thoroughly cleansed with an antiseptic solution before surgery. Some of these bacterial cells can be carried into the breast pocket as the implant is inserted into the breast. The theory is that these few bacterial cells produce a reaction that may result in capsular contracture.

Also, some studies show that inserting implants through the areola results in higher rates of nipple numbness. This is because it is impossible to avoid cutting the nerves around the nipple during this procedure.

Lastly, the areolar approach may decrease the chances of a woman's ability to breastfeed. This is because milk ducts run directly around the nipple and an incision through the areola can disrupt these ducts.

In summary, due to the disadvantages associated with this procedure and, in particular, because of the high rate of capsular contracture, leading breast augmentation surgeons no longer recommend inserting implants through the areola.

BREAST CREASE
(OR INFRAMAMMARY CREASE OR INFRAMAMMARY FOLD)

The breast crease is also called the inframammary crease or the infra-mammary fold (IMF). It is located at the bottom portion of the breast where the breast skin attaches to the chest. This fold is more obvious in larger breasts. Regardless of the breast size, however, the fibers that create the inframammary fold are always present.

Inserting breast implants through the breast crease involves making a 1.25-inch incision that will heal in the position of the final inframammary crease. After making the incision, the surgeon creates a subglandular or submuscular pocket, inserts the implant in it, and then closes the incision. The placement of the incision provides the surgeon a high level of control over the pocket and the shaping of the breast.

The multiple advantages of this approach have made it the ideal technique for breast augmentation. Studies have consistently shown inframammary crease breast augmentations have lower rates of complications, such as capsular contracture, nipple numbness, inability to breastfeed, asymmetry, and irregularities, compared to the preceding techniques you've read about in this section.

For most women, the breast-crease scar heals well and is hidden. (See figures 7.4 through 7.7.) This is true even when a woman has very little breast tissue or does not have a visible inframammary crease before surgery. The reason is the implant, even if it is a small one, creates a curvature at the bottom of the breast. The combination of the curvature and the pressure the implant places on the breast tissue pushes down on the fibers of the inframammary crease. As a result, the inframammary crease is enhanced, and the scar falls nicely within it.

The most highly skilled plastic surgeons can predict with a high degree of accuracy the future position of the scar associated with an inframammary breast augmentation. Although doctors can never (and as a result should never) guarantee a scar's position, they will

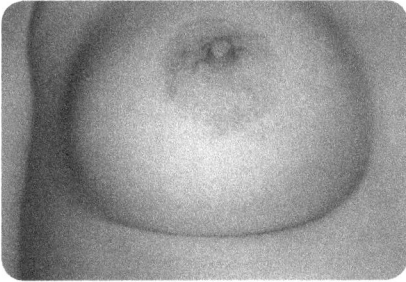

FIGURE 7.4. An example of the incision under the breast crease. As you can see, the scar is hidden within the fold of the breast.

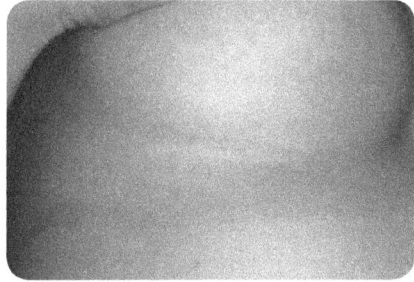

FIGURE 7.5. This is the same patient as in figure 7.4. She is holding her breast up to reveal the scar. As you can see, the scar is barely visible and is designed to fall in the natural inframammary fold (IMF)/ breast crease.

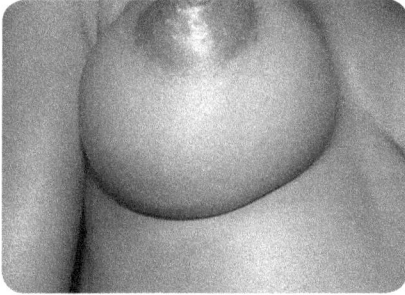

FIGURE 7.6. Another example of the IMF scar in a darker skin person. The scar is hidden under the fold of the breast.

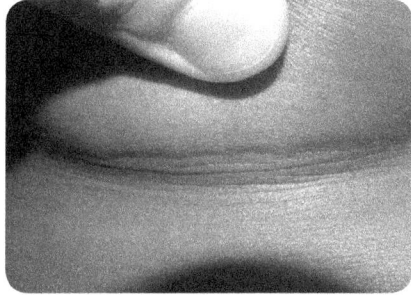

FIGURE 7.7. This is the same patient as in figure 7.6. My thumb is holding the bottom of her breast up. The camera is zoomed in and is tilted up to show the scar. As you can see, the scar is barely visible. It looks like a natural crease in the breast fold.

use their experience as well as measuring tools to make their scar assessment. The scar associated with an inframammary breast augmentation, when planned properly, is superior to all other incision locations. It is not visible in clothing, nor is it visible when viewed from the front, with or without a bra. On the other hand, an areolar incision will *always* be visible from the front without a bra, no matter how well it heals—even a very fine line of an areolar scar will be noticeable when the breast is seen without a bra.

An inframammary scar is hidden, even when you lie on your back. This is because the natural position of the breasts will cause the tissue to fold where the crease is and, therefore, where the scar is. In fact, the inframammary scar is usually only visible when the breast is physically held up and observed from below.

In summary, because of the long list of advantages and the low number of complications compared to the three other incision locations, the inframammary fold technique has become the breast-augmentation standard.

Scar Healing Variations

As the saying goes, "Every rule has an exception." Although I've described the inframammary incision location as the best option for most patients and I've pointed out the many drawbacks of areolar incision procedures, a select group of women may benefit from an areolar incision.

Certain populations of women tend to produce dark scars. These include women of color, such as African American, Asian, and Latina women. While experience has taught me that scars for these women eventually lighten and heal just as well as for other ethnic groups, the healing process is often longer. For example, many women require six months for their scars to considerably fade. But women who are likely to produce dark scars may need twelve to eighteen months to experience a similar result. For these women, they may opt for an areolar incision so they can avoid a longer scar-healing process.

When my patients and I evaluate the benefits and drawbacks of the different incision locations, including the possibility of a lengthy scar-healing process for certain groups of women, most still opt for the inframammary fold incision. For them, the overall benefits of the inframammary fold incision far outweigh its drawbacks. And I agree with them 100 percent.

Summary

- There are four incision location options: the bellybutton (or umbilicus), the armpit (or axilla), the nipple (or areola), and the breast crease (or inframammary crease or inframammary fold) at the bottom of the breast.

- The farther away the incision is from the breast, the more difficult it is for the surgeon to control the results.

- The inframammary incision has been proven to be the best and safest option for breast augmentation.

At this point, you've learned everything you need to know about implants, placement, and incision options. In the next chapter, we will discuss everything you will need to do before the day of surgery.

Breast Augmentation Myths

> My friend had her implants inserted through the bellybutton, and her results look good, so I should go for it too.

No! Every surgery, even the most minor, has risks associated with it. So any anecdotal information, such as your friend's experience or that of any other woman you know or have read about online, should not inform your decision. Your body has features that are particular to it, so your aim should be to receive the best procedure based on your body type, your preferences, and a thorough assessment of each procedure's strengths and weaknesses.

In order to create great results, your surgeon must develop a custom plan that maximizes the chances you'll experience the outcome you seek and minimizes risk and the chances you'll have an unsatisfactory result.

In and of itself, a breast augmentation is a highly complicated procedure—more so when you add the complexity of inserting an implant through the bellybutton or armpit, which decreases a surgeon's ability to see the precise location of the implant, control the implant's position, and shape the breast.

This doesn't mean all patients should avoid a breast augmentation performed through the bellybutton or armpit. But such strategies do increase risks. Think about it in the following terms:

Imagine seven out of ten patients successfully underwent a through-the-bellybutton breast augmentation. That means three patients had an unsatisfactory result. Do you want to run the risk of being one of those three unhappy women?

Top surgeons aim for great results ten out of ten times, and they're able to consistently perform at the highest level possible. One way they accomplish this is through using strategies that have a proven track record for safety and great outcomes—the inframammary incision is one example of this.

An inframammary incision will produce an unsightly scar.

This is the top concern I receive from patients when we discuss the pros and cons of the inframammary incision location. But experience has taught me this technique provides the least noticeable scar of all the incision options patients have.

This is because the fold isn't visible when you're nude. On the other hand, the bellybutton scar is visible whenever the bellybutton is exposed—even if the scar is impeccably designed. Next, the armpit scar often heals darkly because of the presence of hair follicles and sweat glands in the underarm area. In some patients, the darkness can be quite noticeable when they raise their arms wearing sleeveless clothing, such as a tank top, a strapless dress, or a swimsuit. Lastly, the areolar scar, even when it heals perfectly, always leaves a faint line, which is always visible around the nipple.

The inframammary scar is the only one that can be hidden at all times. It is only visible when the breast is lifted and viewed from below. Under most circumstances, the breast's curvature will always hide the scar when you're standing or even lying on your back.

I tend to form keloid scars, so I'm at a higher risk
of scarring.

The main part of this myth is that most people do not have **keloid scars** or the tendency to develop them. What is a keloid scar? It is a rare skin disorder in which the scar tissue continues to grow and widen beyond the borders of the original incision or injury. Keloids spread wildly out of proportion compared to the original incision or laceration. Although many people think they have keloid scars, very few individuals actually have them.

In this case of mistaken identity, what most people do have is a hypertrophic scar. "Hyper" means "more," and "trophic" means "growth." These scars are often dark and raised. Their unsightly appearance may have resulted from a prior surgery or accident.

A scar may become hypertrophic for many reasons. First, if the scar results from an injury, this means it didn't come from a controlled situation, so there was no way to design the scar from the start. This is not the case with elective breast augmentation surgery.

Second, the laceration that caused the scar may be irregular in shape or depth or both. Unless the edges of the laceration are aligned properly, meaning that every point on a cut is matched to its counterpart on the other side of the cut, the scar may not heal well. This is common with scars created by an injury or non-cosmetic surgery.

Third, hypertrophic scars are often caused by tension. Incisions made on the top of or near joints, such as the knee or elbow, are prone to movement or pulling. Because of the constant pulling on the incision's edges, the scar tends to be larger than it would otherwise be if it were on top of a location that wasn't prone to movement or pulling. In the case of the inframammary crease, it experiences minimal, if any, tension.

Lastly, incisions may create hypertrophic scars if they are repaired in just one layer. This means sutures secured only the skin's most superficial surface. Meanwhile, the deeper skin structures were left unrepaired. This often occurs with non-cosmetic surgical procedures, including appendectomies, C-sections, gallbladder removal, and more. The reason is largely practical: The doctor's focus was on treating an underlying medical condition (appendicitis or inflammation of the gall bladder, for example). While the technique the doctor uses to close the incision is safe, the approach emphasizes function over how the closing of the incision will look once healed. This points to an important difference between non-plastic surgeons and plastic surgeons. On one hand, non-plastic surgeons often place a low priority on designing a scar. On the other hand, plastic surgeons focus on aligning scars as perfectly as possible.

Thus, previous experiences you may have had with scars related to accidents and non-cosmetic surgical procedures don't apply to scars associated with breast augmentation because minimizing scars is one of a plastic surgeon's top priorities in a breast augmentation. This includes making an incision and closing it in a way that avoids hypertrophic scars. The bottom line is to resist the temptation to compare any non-cosmetic surgery scar to one you'll receive after a breast augmentation.

CHAPTER 8

PREOPERATIVE PREPARATION

In this chapter, you'll learn:

- essential issues you must address before surgery;

- what steps you must complete before surgery to make sure your surgery and recovery run smoothly.

Real Conversations

It was Monday morning, and Nicole had just phoned Dr. Williams's office to set up her initial consultation. She was thrilled she was able to schedule an appointment with the plastic surgeon for the next day. The timing was perfect—she had the week off from work, and she knew that once she returned to the office, she wouldn't be able to take off any more time for the next few months. So her plans for the week were as follows:

- Attend the consultation on Tuesday.
- Have the breast augmentation performed on Thursday.

• Return to work the next week.

On Tuesday, Nicole's appointment with Dr. Williams went smoothly. After she left the exam room, she met with Alexis, Dr. Williams's patient coordinator.

"When would you like to schedule your surgery?" Alexis asked.

"I only have this week off, so can I schedule it this Thursday?" Nicole asked.

"Whoa!" said Alexis. "That's only two days away. We need to take care of quite a few items the day before surgery, and it will definitely be a stretch for you to complete everything by tomorrow."

Alexis explained that Nicole needed routine blood tests done before Thursday. It was already 4:00 p.m., and the blood lab would be closing shortly. Nicole also had to fill out a significant amount of paperwork, obtain prescription medication, and complete several other pre-op items. The news both surprised and disappointed her.

"I didn't know how much I had to take care of beforehand. I guess my surgery can't happen this week," Nicole said.

"We can certainly try our best. But in all honesty, we may need to schedule your breast augmentation for another week," Alexis said.

Alexis also described the recovery time Nicole would require. She hadn't factored this into her initial calculation. Overall, she realized she had underestimated the time she would need and the effort she would have to give for her breast augmentation.

Introduction

You may experience moments in your life when a surgical procedure must happen and you have no time to prepare. But barring these exceptional and urgent circumstances, when it comes to any major surgery you undergo, you should always allow for the proper amount of time to prepare and recover. In Nicole's case, she initially treated her surgery as if it were the fast-food equivalent of a major medical procedure. The reality is breast augmentation is a serious operation that should never be taken lightly or rushed.

No doubt, a breast augmentation is for cosmetic reasons. But your health and well-being should be your and your surgeon's top priority. This means a positive surgical outcome is a team effort. In this chapter, you'll learn the role you'll play and responsibilities you'll have in order to experience a flawless surgery and recovery.

After the Consultation

Previously, we explored your initial consultation in depth. After you meet with the doctor, the patient coordinator will guide you through the remainder of your appointment. He or she will cover the following essential topics:

- Financing

- Scheduling

- Consent forms

- Laboratory tests

- Preoperative instructions

- Surgery-day preparation

In the next section, we'll explore each of these.

Financing: The Process and Your Options

Most patients find it helpful to make financial arrangements prior to the consultation. In other words, before meeting with the surgeon, they have already determined how they will pay for their breast augmentation. We briefly touched on the financial aspects of your surgery in chapter 1, when you learned about the importance of establishing a budget.

As you read previously, prices for breast augmentation vary greatly. Factors that influence the final cost include the city in which your procedure is performed and the surgeon's reputation. If you're interested in inquiring about costs with your prospective surgeon's office, I recommend you do this during your initial call when you're scheduling your appointment. You'll most likely receive a range of surgical prices. You'll use this information to make sure the doctor you're planning to meet is within your budget. Otherwise, you'll be wasting precious time meeting with surgeons who are beyond your budget. (Also, remember that some doctors charge for the initial consultation.)

Next, most offices require a deposit to schedule a date for your breast augmentation. And because doctors are often booked weeks in advance as far as surgeries are concerned, being able to submit a deposit right away will allow you to secure a surgical day as soon as possible. The remaining balance is usually due between one to two weeks before surgery. This period between payments will allow you to make financial arrangements for the final amount.

If you seek third-party support to help pay for your breast augmentation, many companies finance cosmetic-related procedures. Most of these businesses have websites where you can apply online. Care Credit and Prosper Healthcare Lending are two such companies. Before you sign a credit agreement, make sure you understand the loan's terms and interest rates.

If you're financing your breast augmentation, taking care of this before the consultation will save you time. With that said, you can sometimes wait until you meet with the surgeon's patient coordinator.

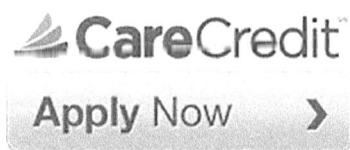

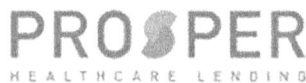

Most doctors' offices have relationships with credit companies and are able to help you through the online application process.

But keep in mind being approved for financing prior to your appointment will allow you to avoid the risks and headaches associated with being declined online if you apply at the doctor's office. By taking care of your payment method in advance, before you meet the doctor, you'll know for certain you've been approved and you'll be able to schedule your surgery without delay. This leads us to the next topic.

Scheduling: Before, During, and After

When it comes to timelines, I always recommend patients plan ahead in order to fully understand how events related to their surgery will unfold. This will ensure you'll have plenty of time to complete all your required pre-surgery to-do tasks. For example, you'll have to fill out a significant amount of paperwork after you've scheduled your surgery. Most patients decide to return to the office on another day to complete this. In my office, we refer to this as the "pre-op appointment."

This step may last from one to two hours, depending on how many follow-up questions you may have. For example, consent paperwork, in and of itself, usually requires only a few minutes to read and sign. But in my experience, when patients come back to fill out paperwork, they have new questions associated with the procedure, and many of them are related to risks associated with the surgery. Asking multiple questions and receiving answers will lengthen the visit. In other words, the total time you'll need largely depends on what questions you would like to have answered. Thus, you'll need to factor this into your overall timeline.

Next, the most significant aspect of scheduling is determining your operation start time. The time of day you must arrive at the doctor's office on surgery day varies. As you learned earlier, most doctors' surgery schedules—and in particular physicians in high

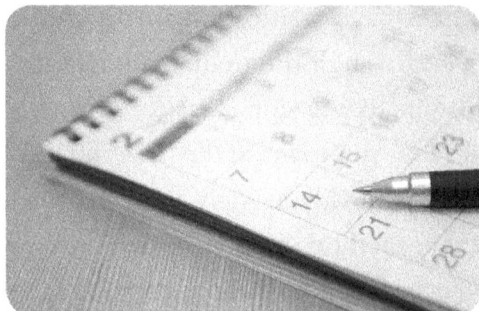

demand—fill up quickly. So the sooner you schedule your appointment after your initial consultation, the more likely you'll be able to book it relatively soon and on a day and time that you prefer most.

In the case of my practice, most people prefer to have their surgery done in the morning. Specifically, they seek to be the first surgery of the day. Reasons include wanting to evade mid-morning and afternoon traffic to Beverly Hills and a preference to avoid going too long without eating (patients aren't allowed to eat or drink anything after midnight the night before their breast augmentation).

As the surgeon's schedule is filled, later times are given to subsequent patients. Therefore, the more in advance you schedule a surgery, the more likely you will be scheduled early in the day.

Once your surgery is done, you'll need to take time off from work or school. How many days will you need? In general, you should allot a minimum of four to five days of recovery after surgery. Taking five to seven days off, however, is ideal. The exact amount of time you'll require depends on many factors, including the type of work you do. During your initial consultation, your surgeon should let you know how much time off you should plan.

Around one week after surgery, you'll have a postoperative visit with your doctor. By this point, many patients are able to drive themselves to this appointment—although most patients feel more comfortable having someone else take them. After this first postoperative appointment, you'll most likely have several more check-ups that will occur over the following months. These later visits are optional and can be scheduled at your convenience.

In chapter 11, we'll explore the recovery process in more depth.

Consent Forms: Taking Your Patient Role Seriously

As you've already learned in this chapter, part of the paperwork that must be completed prior to surgery is surgical consent forms. These outline the risks and benefits associated with your breast augmentation surgery. I can't stress enough the importance you must place in reading every word carefully in order to gain a solid understanding of what your surgery involves. Doing so is one of your most important responsibilities as a well-informed patient. We'll take a deeper look into consent forms in chapter 10.

Laboratory Tests: Required Blood Work

Before any major surgery you undergo, routine blood tests are usually required. Their purpose is to alert the surgeon of any potential issues you may have that can compromise your safety during your operation or your recovery afterwards. In my office, the tests we routinely order are as follows:

- Blood chemistry panel

- Complete blood count

- Coagulation profile

- Serum pregnancy test

- Other blood tests

A **blood chemistry panel** measures the level of vital chemicals in your blood, such as sodium and potassium. Taking these

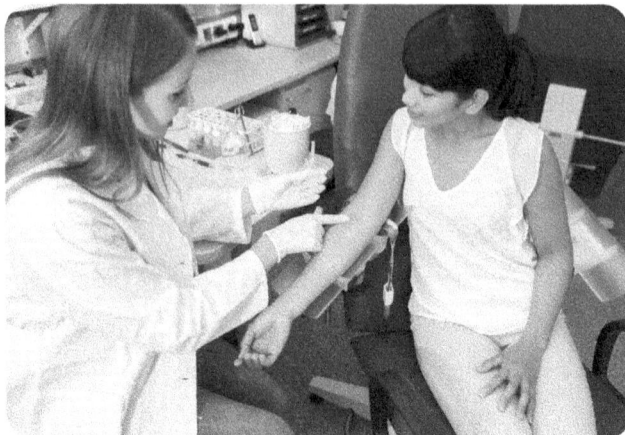

measurements is important because some patients can have hazard-
ously low or high concentrations of chemicals in their body. Depending on what a patient's level is, some women may need additional
treatment to restore their values to normal levels before surgery.
Fortunately, abnormal results are extremely rare.

Another routine test is the **complete blood count**. This measures
the levels of specific cells, such as those that carry oxygen (red blood
cells) and those that are responsible for blood clotting (platelets). If the
concentration of these cells is too low, you may need certain treatments
to increase your level to safe amounts. Similar to blood chemistry pan-
els, abnormal results from complete blood count tests is rare.

A **coagulation profile** measures your blood's ability to clot. This
is important because if your clotting ability is compromised, you will
more likely develop excessive bleeding after surgery. The good news
is patients rarely have any issue with their clotting mechanism.

All patients must also take a **serum pregnancy test**. The
"serum" in a serum pregnancy test refers to your blood, which is
required to perform the test. In addition, on the day of surgery, you
must undergo a second pregnancy test. In this case, a simpler urine
pregnancy test is sufficient.

The role of all blood work is to ensure your safety. Fortunately, since most women seeking breast augmentation are relatively young and healthy, rarely do doctors see abnormalities in any of their patients' blood tests. If any are found, you will be referred to the appropriate medical specialist to receive further evaluation prior to being able to move forward with your breast augmentation.

Preoperative Instructions: What to Do and What to Avoid

Now that you've scheduled your surgery, filled out all consent forms, and received the green light from your blood work for your breast augmentation, it's time to prepare for your big day! In this section, we'll explore other important to-do items on your list that will ensure your operation goes as smoothly as possible.

You'll usually receive a list of what to avoid before surgery. On this list are aspirin; alcohol-containing beverages; various other medications, nutritional supplements, and herbs; and cigarettes and other nicotine-containing products.

Aspirin and aspirin-containing medications interfere with blood clotting and have been associated with increased bleeding during and after surgery. Thus, you want to avoid any aspirin or aspirin-containing medications for at least two weeks prior to surgery. Alcohol is also known to interfere with clotting. So you must stop consuming

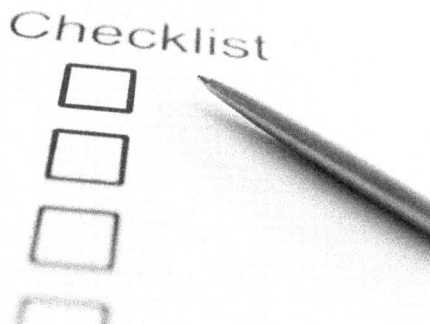

alcohol for about a week before your operation.

Furthermore, you should avoid taking various other medications, as well as nutritional and herbal supplements. Many of these products can affect heart function, or they can cause dangerous changes in blood pressure or heart rate during surgery.

You must also stop smoking cigarettes or taking other nicotine-containing products because nicotine directly interferes with your body's healing process and is known to increase the likelihood of other complications after surgery. Thus, if you smoke or take nicotine-containing products or do both, be sure to inform your doctor so you can establish a timeline for quitting.

In addition to these items, your doctor should give you a detailed list of other "must avoid" items, as well as "must do" ones. This includes instructions highlighting what you need to do the night before and the day of your surgery. For example, you're typically advised to not eat or drink anything after midnight the day before your surgery. This is to ensure you have no food or water in your stomach that you can possibly regurgitate during your procedure. Overall, make sure you review all the items on your doctor's list in order to experience the best outcome possible.

The day prior to your surgery, most doctors advise patients to pick up a few items. At the top of this list are prescription medications. You'll receive a list of medications to take after your operation. I advise my patients to pick these up the day before their procedure, so they are ready to take them once they arrive home after their breast augmentation.

Next, I recommend my patients stock up on groceries and snacks. Your recovery will be much more comfortable and easier with a well-stocked refrigerator.

Also, don't forget to download movies and books to enjoy during your recovery. After all, you'll be resting in bed and on the couch for the next few days. So curling up with good movies and books will make your recovery a more pleasant experience

Lastly, you must arrange to have an adult pick you up after surgery and care for you after. Patients are not allowed to leave the surgical facility unless someone is available to care for them. You should make arrangements with this person far in advance, since she or he will need to take time off from work or school.

Surgery-Day Preparation

On the day of surgery, I recommend you wear loose-fitting and comfortable clothes. Drawstring sweatpants and sweaters with a zipper front are best. Wearing these will make it much easier for you to dress and undress after your surgery is completed.

Next, make sure to remove any jewelry or piercings that can become snagged on surgical fabrics, such as the gowns you will be wearing and the curtains around your operating room bed. Injuries to your skin can result when jewelry or piercings get caught on these fabrics. Even worse, metal jewelry and piercings may interfere with the electricity that powers surgical instruments. Metal piercings and jewelry on the body have also been known to conduct electricity during surgery. The electricity running through a piercing or item of jewelry can cause the metal to heat up, and this can burn your surrounding skin.

Summary

- Important issues that need to be addressed before your surgery include financial payments, scheduling, informed consents, laboratory tests, preoperative instructions, and surgery-day preparations.

- There are several steps for each of these that must be completed in advance in order to make sure your surgery day runs smoothly.

A COMPREHENSIVE GUIDE TO BREAST AUGMENTATION

The next chapter will cover essential information you should know before surgery. This includes an overview of the most common complications associated with breast augmentation. By reviewing this information, you will ensure that you are as informed as possible before signing any consent forms.

Breast Augmentation Myths

> I can have an initial consultation and the breast augmentation both completed in the same week.

Although scheduling and undergoing surgery within a few days after an initial consultation is possible, this isn't common, and I don't recommend it for multiple reasons.

First of all, breast augmentation is a major medical procedure. Thus you should give yourself enough time to research, consider, and process the multiple decisions you must make regarding your surgery. As I do with my own patients, I encourage you to thoroughly consider the pros and cons associated with your surgery. The outcome of a breast augmentation is permanent, so it is not a decision you should ever rush or take lightly.

Second, you must complete a long list of to-do items prior to your surgery. These include securing financing, filling out in-depth paperwork, undergoing routine blood tests, scheduling the recovery time you need, and arranging for outside help after surgery.

Most of my patients require a few weeks to check off all items on their to-do list. Thus, the more time you give yourself, the more likely your must-do tasks will be completed to the highest degree possible.

In the end, every step you complete in this extensive process has the following objectives: to put your smooth and speedy recovery at

134

the forefront, ensure your safety, avoid medical complications, and create the environment necessary for your surgeon to perform at his or her best.

CHAPTER 9

INFORMED CONSENT

In this chapter, you'll learn:

- potential risks associated with breast augmentation;

- advanced techniques I use during surgery to avoid complications.

Real Conversations

"These are your informed-consent forms," I said as Courtney, my patient coordinator, handed the paperwork to Rebecca. "They review the risks, benefits, and alternatives you discussed with me during your appointment. Read these carefully, and if you have any questions, I'll be happy to answer them."

For Rebecca, receiving the information marked one more step closer to having the breasts she had wanted for so long. She looked forward to the surgery more than ever. When she arrived home, Rebecca began reviewing the forms.

"Capsular contracture, asymmetry, scarring . . . all these risks are making me nervous. I thought this was going to be an easy procedure. I think I need to meet with Dr. Diaz again," she told herself.

When I met with Rebecca again, I addressed her list of concerns.

"Every surgery has risks, but in the hands of a skilled and careful surgeon, they are low," I said.

The information I provided her during our appointment diminished her anxieties. Afterwards, she submitted her signed consent forms.

"I was so nervous after reading the paperwork you gave me. Now that Dr. Diaz has answered my questions, I'm excited to move forward," she told Courtney.

Introduction

Breast augmentation is one of the safest of all surgical procedures. And as a surgeon who has performed countless breast augmentations, I can confidently say that by upholding the highest medical standards possible, the operation is extremely safe. With that said, it is surgery nonetheless. Thus, as is the case with all operations, both major and minor, unexpected side effects or complications can always happen. After all, even removing a small mole has risks!

So before you read on, keep in mind that when you work with a top-notch board-certified plastic surgeon, the risks that appear in this chapter are unlikely to occur. But, as a plastic surgeon who upholds the highest standards of safety and patient communication, it's important that I point these out to you.

Some risks are common to all surgeries (breast augmentations, as well as cosmetic and non-cosmetic procedures). And some are associated with the implants themselves. Meanwhile, other risks are entirely subjective. In other words, they relate to your satisfaction or dissatisfaction with your appearance, even if the procedure itself was

INFORMED CONSENT –
AUGMENTATION MAMMAPLASTY WITH SILICONE GEL-FILLED IMPLANTS

INSTRUCTIONS

This is an informed-consent document that has been prepared to help inform you concerning augmentation mammaplasty surgery with silicone gel-filled implants, its risks, as well as alternative treatment(s).

It is important that you read this information carefully and completely. Please initial each page, indicating that you have read the page and sign the consent for surgery as proposed by your plastic surgeon and agreed upon by you.

GENERAL INFORMATION

In November, 2006, silicone gel-filled breast implant devices were approved by the United States Food and Drug Administration (FDA) for use in breast augmentation and reconstruction.

Augmentation mammaplasty is a surgical operation performed to enlarge the female breasts for a number of reasons:

- To enhance the body contour of a woman, who for personal reasons feels that her breast size is too small.
- To correct a loss in breast volume after pregnancy.
- To balance breast size, when there exists a significant difference between the size of the breasts.
- To restore breast shape after partial or total loss of the breasts from various conditions.
- To correct a failure of breast development due to a severe breast abnormality.
- To correct or improve results of existing breast implants for cosmetic or reconstructive reasons.

Breast implant surgery is contraindicated in women with untreated breast cancer or pre-malignant breast disorders, active infection anywhere in the body, or individuals who are currently pregnant or nursing.

Individuals with a weakened immune system (currently receiving chemotherapy or drugs to suppress the immune system), conditions that interfere with blood clotting or wound healing, or have reduced blood supply to the breast tissue from prior surgery or radiation therapy treatments may be at greater risk for complications and poor surgical outcome.

Silicone breast implants are approved by the FDA for use in women who are at least 22 years of age. Women who meet this age criteria may utilize the silicone implants for cosmetic breast augmentation or for revision surgery to correct or improve results of earlier cosmetic breast augmentation. There is no age restriction on breast reconstruction procedures to restore breast shape after cancer, trauma, or severe breast abnormalities.

Breast enlargement is accomplished by inserting a breast implant either behind the breast tissue, or partially or completely under the chest muscles. Incisions are made to keep scars as inconspicuous as possible, usually under the breast, around a portion of areola, or in the armpit. According to the FDA it is not recommended to use the peri-umbilical approach to insert gel-filled implants. Breast implants may be manufactured in a variety of shapes, sizes, and with either smooth or textured surfaces. The method of implant selection and size, along with surgical approach for inserting and positioning breast implants will depend on your preferences, your anatomy and your surgeon's recommendation. The shape and size of the breasts prior to surgery will influence both the recommended treatment and the final results. If the breasts are not the same size or shape before surgery, it is unlikely that they will be completely symmetrical afterward.

Conditions which involve sagging of the breast or diminished skin tone (stretch marks) may require additional surgical procedures (breast lift) to reposition the nipple and areola upward and to remove loose skin.

Patients undergoing augmentation mammaplasty surgery must consider the following:

- Breast augmentation or reconstruction with silicone gel-filled implants may not be a one time surgery.
- Breast implants of any type are not considered lifetime devices. They cannot be expected to last forever. You will likely require future surgery for implant replacement or removal.

100 percent successful from a safety point of view.

In this chapter, I'll provide an overview of the main risks associated with breast augmentation surgery. This chapter is broad in scope, so make sure to discuss specific risks in detail during your consultation with your plastic surgeon.

General Risks

In this section, you'll learn about the following general risks associated with breast augmentation:

- Dissatisfaction with size

- Asymmetry

- Unsightly scarring

- Bleeding and hematoma

- Infection

- Decreased nipple sensation

- Inability to breastfeed

- Cancer and detection

DISSATISFACTION WITH SIZE

As the saying goes, "Beauty is in the eye of the beholder." When it comes to breast augmentation, this is especially true. Ultimately, the aesthetic results of cosmetic surgery are always subjective. In other words, the evaluation of a result varies depending on who is evaluating it.

For instance, let's say Katherine and Melissa are the same height and weight and have the same body shape and breast measurements. They both undergo a breast augmentation and obtain the same type and size implants. After Katherine's recovery, she looks in the mirror and thinks her breasts are too big. Meanwhile, Melissa, whose breasts look similar to Katherine's, is frustrated that her new breast size is still too small.

This illustrates one way in which a patient may not be pleased with her surgical outcome. In your case, you may stare at your body in a full-length mirror after your surgery and wish your breasts were bigger, or you may be worried they are too large. Or you may, for

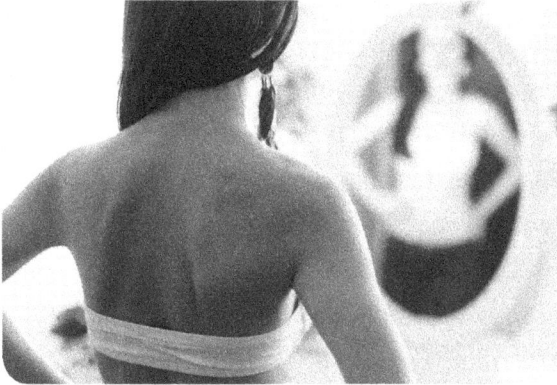

any number of reasons, not like their overall appearance—even though the result looks perfect to everyone else. A key way to avoid this unfortunate predicament is to have an exhaustive and thorough consultation with your plastic surgeon prior to your procedure. By working closely with a top surgeon, he or she will identify and assess your needs by using the latest technology, as well as his or her experience and extensive track record of performing breast augmentations.

For instance, as you read previously, in my office I use the Vectra 3D imaging system. Only a few surgeons in the world have this. For review, the Vectra 3D system takes multiple high-resolution photos of your breasts and converts them to three-dimensional images. The system then takes your breast images and provides simulations of what your breasts will look like with the implants you've selected. From there, you'll have ample time to evaluate your results and decide which implants will best match the overall look you seek. Using this system has allowed me to achieve great results with extremely high patient satisfaction.

ASYMMETRY

Every feature of our body is **asymmetric**, which means the right side is slightly different from the left side. Usually, the differences are so small it is not very noticeable. For instance, the right ear might be a little larger than the left ear. Or the right arm might be slightly longer than the left arm. In other words, from top to bottom, the left and right sides of our bodies are not perfectly symmetrical.

So when it comes to your breasts, every woman's breasts are slightly different on each side. In this way, you can think of your two breasts as "sisters, not twins." Indeed, some women's breasts are more symmetrical than others. But even breasts that look perfectly symmetrical, upon close inspection, never are. Meanwhile, other women's asymmetry is more apparent—their breasts vary greatly in position or shape or size or any combination of the preceding. It is interesting to note that few people are able to notice these asymmetries on their own bodies. In fact, even women with significant asymmetry of their breasts are surprised when I point this out to them.

The truth is that the more different the breasts appear before surgery, the more likely asymmetry will continue after. Your surgeon can take steps to correct asymmetry during the procedure, such as using one size implant in one breast and another size implant in the other, as well as manipulating the breast-implant position. But even if asymmetries are addressed, some differences will persist.

A highly experienced plastic surgeon knows how to identify your specific breast asymmetries and determine the best course of action to correct them. He or she will review your surgical options with you during your consultation.

UNSIGHTLY SCARRING

As you read previously in this book, a plastic surgeon's ability to design a scar that is as undetectable as possible is a significant sign of his or her superb training and skill. Plastic surgeons spend a great deal of their training learning how to design scars that are thin, faint, and barely noticeable. So the good news is that for most patients, a well-designed scar will heal incredibly well and will be nearly invisible.

If you currently have a post-surgery scar that bothers you, keep in mind that most likely a non-plastic surgeon performed your previous operation. This means that scar will never look as good as one a plastic surgeon will design. So if you've been left with an unsightly scar from a prior surgery, this doesn't signal you'll have an unsightly scar after your breast augmentation.

At the same time, there is always the possibility that your scar will heal in an unsightly way. As mentioned previously, some people are prone to forming darker and thicker scars. These include women of color, such as African American, Asian, and Latina patients. But even among women who are prone to scars, they usually fade and improve over time.

Regardless of your skin coloring or ethnic background, all scars, even perfectly designed ones, will take up to a year to fully heal. Specifically, all scars are slightly red and raised during the first few weeks post-surgery. After a month or two, the scar will begin to fade. Eventually, it will be barely noticeable. But to reach that stage, patients usually need to wait six months to a year.

While unsightly scar healing is rare, if for whatever reason, you're unhappy with how it looks, other treatments can minimize a scar's appearance. Today, cutting-edge skin-care products, injections, and lasers can effectively diminish a scar's overall profile.

BLEEDING AND HEMATOMA

Any kind of surgery, even the most minor, will cause bleeding—this is normal and should be expected. But in rare cases, excessive bleeding may occur during or after surgery. If this happens, additional surgery or transfusions may be required.

In some instances, bleeding may take place after surgery, and the blood may accumulate slowly in the breast pocket. As it collects, it can result in a **hematoma**, which is a collection of blood as a result of a ruptured blood vessel. In this case, the hematoma is inside the breast pocket. Once a hematoma is formed, your surgeon must drain it. With that said, when your surgeon follows a meticulously developed surgical plan, the risks of excessive bleeding or hematoma formation are very low.

INFECTION

With any surgery, infection is possible. Fortunately, overall breast augmentation infection rates are extremely low. In the unlikely event you do experience an infection, it will most likely be minor. For example, the incision site can develop a superficial infection. This is typically easy to treat with antibiotics and basic wound care.

For serious infection cases, more aggressive treatment may be required. This may include a prolonged antibiotic course or hospitalization or additional surgery or any combination of these three.

It is very rare for infection to occur when the breast augmentation is performed by an experienced and skilled, board-certified plastic surgeon. Top surgeons, like myself, maintain strict sterility throughout the procedure. For instance, in my case, I take extra precautions, such as using a Keller Funnel to insert the implant and washing the skin around the breast several times during the operation to prevent any infection. As a result, I've maintained an impeccable safety track record.

DECREASED NIPPLE SENSATION

Any breast surgery may affect nipple sensation. This is in large part because the nerves that allow for nipple sensation are not visible to the naked eye. Thus it is impossible for a surgeon to completely avoid damaging the nerves during your operation. Fortunately, decreased nipple sensation is unlikely—even if the surgery affects some nerves.

But keep in mind some insertion points are riskier than others. For example, studies have shown that nipple numbness is more likely to occur when implants are inserted around the nipple or areola because this insertion point is more likely to injure the nerves around the nipple. This is one reason, among others, I usually advise against inserting implants through the nipple and instead recommend making the incision below the breast in the breast crease.

INABILITY TO BREASTFEED
Most women are able to breastfeed after breast augmentation. This is especially true for women who have had breast implants inserted under the breast in the breast crease because inserting implants in this position avoids cutting into the milk ducts, which allows breastfeeding to occur.

On the other hand, inserting implants through the nipple or areola requires cutting into the milk ducts, and this increases the risk you will not be able to breastfeed.

Regardless of the incision you choose, however, there is always some risk that you may have a problem breastfeeding. A very small percentage of women are unable to breastfeed at all. In other cases, women are able to produce milk but in limited amounts, which means they'll need to supplement with formula. Fortunately, the vast majority of women are able to breastfeed normally after breast augmentation.

An increased likelihood of being able to breastfeed without problems is one reason I recommend inserting implants under the breast in the breast crease.

CANCER AND DETECTION
"Will breast augmentation put me at a higher risk for breast cancer?" patients often ask me.

This is a common concern, and you'll find a significant amount of research that has focused on the relationship between breast implants and breast cancer. In fact, the use of silicone implants was temporarily halted for several years to specifically find if any correlation existed. The good news is no data currently suggests breast implants increase breast cancer risk. This is true for both saline and silicone implants.

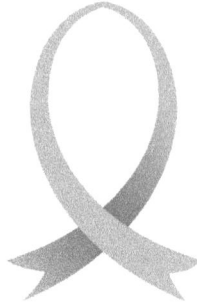

In addition, studies also show that implants do not interfere with mammograms or breast cancer detection. This is especially true for implants placed below the muscle because mammograms and other screening tests are more accurate with submuscular implants. This is one reason I recommend patients place implants below the muscle.

Also, studies have shown that women with implants who develop breast cancer have the same health outcomes as women without implants who develop breast cancer. In other words, both groups required the same amount of time to diagnose and treat their cancers. Furthermore, the rates of survival and being cured are identical for both groups.

Thus you can feel secure knowing your breast implants will not increase your risk of breast cancer or interfere with its detection or treatment. Implants have been exhaustively evaluated, and the research has demonstrated the procedures and the implants themselves are safe.

Risks Associated with Implants

In this section, you'll learn about the following three risks associated with implants:

- Rupture

- Capsular contracture

- Skin wrinkling and rippling

RUPTURE

The latest generation of saline and silicone breast implants are vastly superior to ones manufactured in the past. In fact, to demonstrate their strong and durable design, I'll frequently throw them against a wall or the floor during a consultation. Patients are amazed and reassured when they see the implants remain completely intact. But regardless of how well-built breast implants are, first and foremost, you must realize they are medical devices. And as is the case with all medical devices, breast implants can fail.

So despite the breakthrough advances in implant design and construction, the possibility always exists that they can rupture, even if that likelihood is extremely rare. Sometimes implants can rupture due to a severe injury, such as from a fall from a great height or a serious car accident, or they can rupture for no apparent reason at all. So what happens when an implant ruptures?

If a **saline implant** ruptures, the only symptom you'll most likely experience is the breast with the ruptured implant will appear smaller and smaller over time compared to the breast with the intact implant. It is when you notice shrinking you'll most likely be motivated to make an appointment to meet with your surgeon. In other words, you probably will only observe physical changes to the breast size and not experience any pain or other medical condition.

When a saline implant ruptures, the implant releases the saline fill, and your body absorbs it. The amount of time your body will need to absorb the salt water typically ranges from one to several weeks. Once your doctor has determined your implant has ruptured, he or she will have to replace the broken implant in order to restore your breast's size and shape.

If a **silicone implant** ruptures, you may not notice any change in your breast's size and shape. While you may have read or heard horror stories related to ruptured silicone implants leaking into surrounding breast tissue, these are associated with previous-generation implants that contained a liquid form of silicone.

Today's silicone implants contain silicone gel with a thicker consistency than older models. This means that new implants will stay inside the implant's shell and the scar tissue surrounding the implant. Thus, if a modern silicone implant ruptures, you may not feel or notice any change in your breast. For this reason, very few plastic surgeons would recommend surgery to replace a silicone implant, even if it ruptures. Surgery is only required if the person sees or feels a difference in her breasts. Since this is unlikely, having another surgery is usually not necessary.

Because ruptures in modern silicone implants are so difficult to detect, the Federal Drug Administration (FDA) recommends regular MRI examinations for women with silicone breast implants. This is the only reliable test to determine if a rupture exists. As mentioned previously, this is only a recommendation and is not a requirement. And even if the MRI did show a rupture, most plastic surgeons would not recommend any treatment—particularly if the woman does not feel or see anything different about her breasts. For these reasons, very few women choose to undergo MRIs to detect a rupture in their silicone breast implants or follow the FDA's recommendations for MRIs for silicone breast implants.

CAPSULAR CONTRACTURE

The human body will form scar tissue around any medical device, which includes a breast implant. Under most circumstances, the scar tissue (called a capsule) around an implant is very thin and soft and not noticeable. In some instances, and for reasons not yet fully understood, the scar tissue can become thick and hard. If the condition worsens, the scar tissue will begin to contract and squeeze on the implant, which may cause the breast to appear distorted in shape and to feel very firm. This phenomenon is called capsular contracture (see figure 9.1).

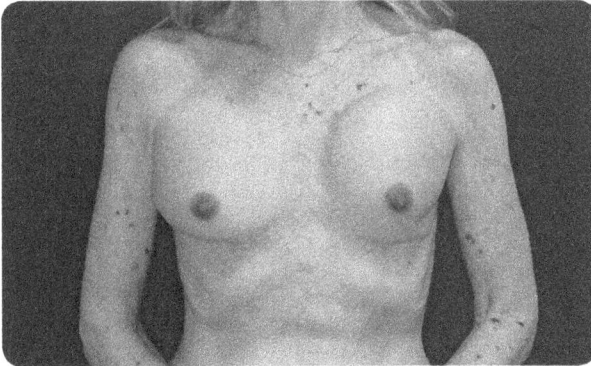

FIGURE 9.1. An example of a patient with capsular contracture of the breasts.

While no one is sure why capsular contracture occurs, what is certain is the chance of it happening ranges from about 1 to 15 percent of women. Some surgeons have a high rate of capsular contracture in their practice, and some have a low rate. For example, over a four-year period, I conducted a study of my patients. I found that among over 1,400 breast augmentations I performed, my patient rate of capsular contracture was only 1 percent, which is the lowest rate possible among all plastic surgeons.

So how do I maintain the industry's lowest rate of capsular contracture? I developed a four-part approach to prevent capsular contracture. This approach was developed as a result of identifying the known conditions that lead to high rates of capsular contracture and directly addressing them.

1. Point of Insertion

Because inserting the implant through the bellybutton, armpit, or nipple-areola increases the likelihood of capsular contracture, I always recommend my patients insert the implant through the crease under the breast.

2. Excessive Bleeding

Because a high degree of bleeding in the breast during surgery increases the likelihood of capsular contracture, I have perfected my surgical approach to diminish bleeding as much as possible. On my website, I have posted videos that show how I prevent excessive bleeding. Go to www.DrJohnDiazBreastAugmentation.com.

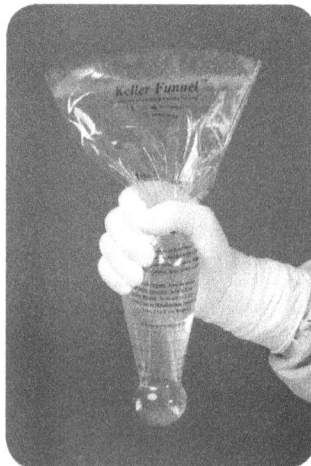

FIGURE 9.2. An implant sleeve called a Keller Funnel.

3. Micro-contamination

Because contamination of the implant or the breast increases the likelihood of capsular contracture, I use a "no-touch" technique.

This includes changing my gloves throughout the surgery; using an implant sleeve, called a Keller Funnel (see figure 9.2), in order to insert the implant; and washing the breast skin multiple times in order to protect the implant and breast from micro contamination. I have posted videos on my website that show my no-touch technique. Go to www.DrJohnDiazBreastAugmentation.com.

4. Implant Placement

Because placing the implant *above* the chest muscle (also called subglandular) has been shown to increase the risk of capsular contracture, I always recommend my patients place the implant *below* the muscle (also called submuscular). One theory why placing an implant below the muscle decreases capsular contracture is this placement prevents scar tissue from thickening and hardening because of muscle movement that occurs over the implant.

By strictly adhering to this four-part approach, my patients experience the lowest possible rates of capsular contracture. But regardless of how many precautions I take, capsular contracture is unavoidable for some patients. In the rare instance it does occur, patients have several effective options to improve it. In very mild cases, you can treat it with oral medications. In severe cases, additional surgery may be required to decrease it. Your board-certified plastic surgeon will review your options with you.

The best way to eliminate capsular contracture is to stop its occurrence before it happens. By working with a doctor whose surgical approach directly addresses it, you'll minimize your risk of experiencing it.

SKIN WRINKLING AND RIPPLING

Skin wrinkling and rippling describes when you can see or feel the implant edges (see figure 9.3). One common reason wrinkling and

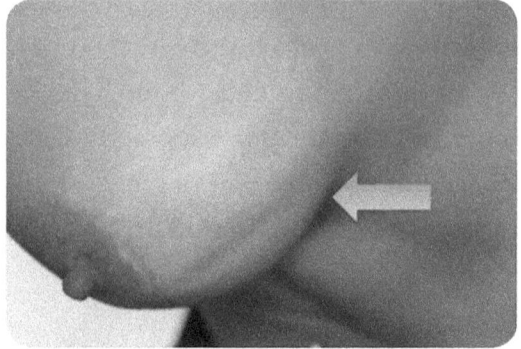

FIGURE 9.3. An example of a patient with rippling. The arrow points to the presence of ripples along the bottom of the patient's breasts.

rippling occurs is many women undergoing breast augmentation have a small amount of breast tissue to begin with. Thus once the implant is in place, only a thin amount of breast tissue will cover it.

One of the advantages of submuscular placement is it provides more cushion over the implant compared to subglandular placement, thereby decreasing the chance of wrinkling and rippling. But even with below-the-muscle placement, the edges of the implant may still have little cushion. This is especially true in the bottom part and side of the breast where the implant edges may be easily seen or felt.

Also, skin wrinkling and rippling are much more common with saline implants. This is one important reason why I recommend silicone implants. Nevertheless, while wrinkling and rippling are less common when silicone implants are used, they may still occur.

Summary

- Breast augmentation, when performed by a board-certified plastic surgeon, is a safe procedure.

- All surgery, no matter how small it is, has potential risks.

- There are numerous advanced techniques a surgeon can use to minimize the risk of complications.

In the next chapter, I will discuss everything you can expect on the day of your surgery.

Breast Augmentation Myths

Surgical complications are always the result of a doctor doing something wrong.

The human body is an incredibly complex and dynamic living structure. And surgery on the human body is equally as complicated. Your doctor must address countless variables and attempt to control every single one of them. Performing successful surgeries frequently, consistently, and predictably is both a challenge and a goal of every top doctor.

Furthermore, within your breasts are millions of blood vessels, nerves, muscle fibers, and other tissues. Surgery alters these structures in ways that aren't always predictable. For example, swelling and scarring may interfere with proper healing and cause unintended changes, such as an irregularity in the contour of the side of the breast or a difference in the appearance of the inframammary scar. In other words, the body is unpredictable—some complications occur even when a surgery is performed perfectly.

No surgeon ever wants a complication. In fact, all outstanding plastic surgeons do everything possible to address potential complications before they ever arise. But no matter how careful a surgeon is, he or she can never guarantee a complication-free result—no matter how much the doctor wishes this were possible!

A top board-certified plastic surgeon strives to achieve perfect results every time. These outstanding doctors implement techniques that minimize risk and maximize positive outcomes before, during, and after surgery. When you work with a foremost surgeon, you can feel confident you'll receive the highest levels of care and results.

CHAPTER 10

THE SURGERY

In this chapter, you'll learn:

- how events will unfold on your big day;

- what the surgery process comprises;

- what to expect after your surgery.

Real Conversations

"My nerves are all over the place!" Michelle told her best friend, Tiffany.

Michelle's breast augmentation was scheduled for the next day. This was the first surgical procedure she had ever undergone, and she was filled with uncertainty about the operation.

"Didn't your doctor tell you what you should expect?" Tiffany asked.

"Not really. It all feels so mysterious," she said.

Michelle was told to show up at the plastic surgeon's office at 6:30 a.m. the next day. But beyond that, she hadn't received additional details regarding what she should be prepared for.

"That's all you were told? No wonder you're nervous. I'd be too," said Tiffany.

Introduction

When I meet with patients looking for a second opinion who have undergone breast augmentation with other surgeons, many of them tell me of experiences similar to Michelle's. They were already nervous about their procedures, and without receiving a detailed explanation of what to expect on surgery day, their tensions ran even higher. Undergoing breast augmentation can be stressful and full of uncertainty. Patients may find themselves asking questions such as, "What will happen pre-op, during surgery, and post-op?" and "How will I feel afterwards?"

But if done right, your surgery doesn't have to be nerve-racking. In fact, it can be a downright positive experience—I know this because my patients tell me this all the time after I've performed their breast augmentations.

My approach is rooted in the following: When women undergo breast augmentation, it's a procedure they've been dreaming of for years. Thus, my goal is to provide my patients an experience that lives up to their expectations. And a big reason my patients don't experience the headaches other women do is the emphasis I place on communication.

All top plastic surgeons realize that knowledge and understanding are essential to decreasing the anxiety associated with the unknown. Thus, part of helping patients maintain peace of mind involves providing a detailed explanation of what to expect on surgery day. As a result, surgery is no longer mysterious and intimidating.

In this chapter, you'll learn the important events that will take place on your big day, from the moment you walk in the door, to the procedure itself, and to your car ride back home. You'll receive the same information I provide my own patients in my practice.

One final introductory note: While all surgeons are trained to provide safe procedures, each surgeon has his or her particular strategy to perform a breast augmentation. This means I cannot describe every surgeon's specific approach. What I can do with 100 percent certainty is describe mine. And this is the process you'll read about in this chapter.

Morning of Surgery

If you're my patient, from the time you arrive for your breast augmentation until the time you leave is about three hours. While the surgery itself takes only about forty-five to sixty minutes, the steps before and after surgery will require additional time. And you'll learn about each step in the following sections.

YOUR ARRIVAL

Breast augmentations usually begin early in the morning. In fact, most doctors start surgeries around 7:30 a.m. This custom has its roots in how hospitals are run. There, surgeries begin at this time. The benefit of an early start is it allows enough time for the surgeon to accomplish everything he or she needs to do.

Regardless of when your surgery is scheduled, you will likely be requested to arrive at the surgical facility an hour before your scheduled surgery time so the surgical staff can prepare you for the procedure.

COMPLETING PAPERWORK

Upon your arrival, my staff will provide you with paperwork to complete. You'll be asked to confirm information regarding how my team will contact you and the family member or friend who will

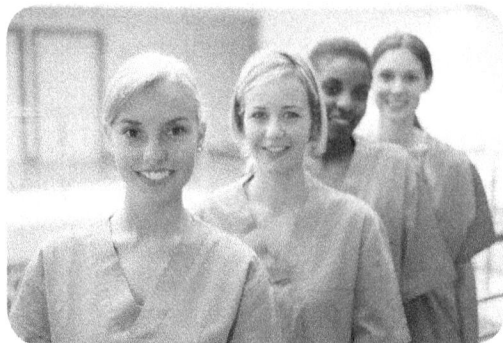

be taking care of you. Also, you'll be provided with forms to review regarding anesthesia and ones that will ask questions about previous medical and surgical treatments you've had. These are similar to what you filled out during previous appointments and are an important step to ensuring all your information is accurate and up to date.

CHANGING ROOM AND PREGNANCY TEST

Once you've filled out all paperwork, you'll be taken to a changing room. In my Beverly Hills office, you'll be provided a locker with key, a gown, and a bag in which to place your belongings.

As you read previously in this book, patients cannot be pregnant prior to surgery. Thus, once you've changed, you must pass a urine test to make sure you're not expecting. A nurse then reviews the test results with you and finalizes any remaining paperwork.

MEET THE ANESTHESIOLOGIST

This is the doctor responsible for administering anesthesia and monitoring your status throughout surgery. Most patients hear the word "anesthesia" and become nervous. They may have been influenced by TV shows and movies that depict patients unintentionally waking up in the middle of surgery. But outside of films and soap operas, regaining consciousness mid-surgery just doesn't happen. Anesthesia is safe and effective, especially if you're healthy and don't suffer from any diseases such as heart or lung problems.

During your meeting with your anesthesiologist, he or she will explain what you'll experience before, during, and after your operation and answer any questions you'll have. Your anesthesiologist will review your medical history to make sure he or she can take the best possible care of you.

MEET YOUR PLASTIC SURGEON

Next, you and I will meet. I will take preoperative photos of your chest. The purpose of these pictures is to document how your breasts look prior to surgery. I then use a soft-tip pen made for marking the skin to outline areas of the breast and the proposed areas of surgery. During this step, I'll spend as much time as you need to ask questions and express concerns. I'll also review any steps you're unclear about.

After you've received all the clarification you need and you're prepared to move forward, you will give your consent to continue. This signals you're ready to start surgery.

Surgery Preparation

In this section, you'll learn how my team and I prepare for your breast augmentation. This includes the following steps:

- Induction of anesthesia

- Prepping the skin

- Draping

- Instrument sets

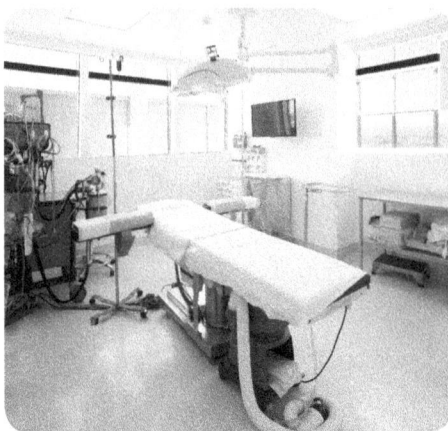

FIGURE 10.1. The operating room.

INDUCTION OF ANESTHESIA

Once you're brought to the operating room, you'll lie down on the operating room bed, which has extensions on the left and right sides so you can rest your arms (see figure 10.1).

The anesthesiologist then inserts an IV into your arm or hand vein. Through this IV, you'll be administered medications.

These medications include several that will relax you and make you feel as comfortable as possible. They also put you in a preliminary sleep stage. Next, a special mask called a "laryngeal mask airway" is inserted into the mouth. Laryngeal refers to the part of the mask that covers your larynx, which is the part of the throat and neck that leads to the lungs. This mask is used to create a seal between the mask and your lungs. Once the seal is made, the anesthesiologist begins to supply your lungs with a mixture of medications that are administered in gas form, which puts you in a deep sleep. When you're in a stable and deep sleep, I will begin the procedure.

Throughout your operation, the anesthesiologist and I work together. He or she closely monitors your heart rate, blood pressure, and the amount of oxygen in your blood stream. The anesthesiologist also analyzes the gas that you exhale through your lungs. All this data is carefully recorded and used to ensure you're receiving the perfect amount of medications necessary to keep you asleep and comfortable during surgery.

In addition to anesthesia, you'll also receive other medications. One is an antibiotic, which will prevent infection. Another is an anti-nausea drug that prevents nausea and vomiting after surgery. You'll also receive pain medications that will make you feel as comfortable as possible. These drugs are administered at the beginning, middle, and end of surgery so that your recovery is as smooth as possible.

PREPPING THE SKIN
This refers to preparing the skin in order to prevent infection. In this process, the chest area is washed with a special hospital-grade antibiotic solution, which kills the bacteria on the skin. This solution is applied and then allowed to dry.

DRAPING
Once the antibiotic solution is dry, drapes made of sterile fabric will cover your entire body with the exception of the breast area. This creates a sterile environment for the breasts.

INSTRUMENT SETS
Once the breasts are covered, a surgical scrub technician, who assists me, prepares a tray with all the surgical instruments I will use. The surgical scrub tech's job is to pass instruments to me throughout your operation. The tray is placed next to the bed, and I'll now begin the breast augmentation.

The Surgical Process

In this section, you'll gain insight into the surgical process I've perfected. For over a decade, I've been performing breast augmentations, and my approach combines proven strategies with my innovative technique. I've also produced high-quality videos that show you how surgery is performed. To see my complete series on YouTube, go to https://www.youtube.com/user/DrJohnDiaz. In this section, we'll cover the following steps:

- Local infiltration

- Incision

- Submuscular plane: sizers and hemostasis

- Re-prepping

- Implants: opening of package, no-touch technique, implant insertion

- Other breast

- Closure of incisions

- Bra placement

LOCAL INFILTRATION

Once the surgical instruments are ready, I inject specific areas of the breast with a solution consisting of epinephrine and lidocaine. Epinephrine is similar to adrenaline, which constricts the blood vessels in the breast tissues. This causes the blood vessels to close, which prevents bleeding during surgery. Lidocaine is a numbing medication that helps prevents you from feeling pain.

INCISION

As you read earlier in this chapter, I use a pen to mark your chest area based on the surgical strategy we've both agreed upon. The lines drawn on your chest area will guide me as I use a scalpel to make the initial incision. Using a scalpel makes the incision as fine as possible.

SUBMUSCULAR PLANE: SIZERS AND HEMOSTASIS

Once the pectoralis muscle (the chest muscle) is exposed, I will then create a submuscular pocket. I do this by entering the space that exists naturally between the muscle and rib cage. Once I've opened and expanded the space, I can insert an implant.

In order for the implant to fit properly, the muscle tissue must be divided at the breast's bottommost part, which is where the breast attaches to the rib cage. This is a must-do step in order to prevent the implant from sitting too high on the chest. Dividing the muscle also allows the implant to fall into place and the breast to relax and settle over time.

Next, I shape the pocket where I'll place the implant. Once I've opened the submuscular space to my satisfaction, the preliminary shaping is done.

I then test the pocket by inserting a **sizer**, which is a temporary implant. I use this to fine-tune the shape and make final decisions about the implant and the breast pocket. I then fill the sizer to the volume we had agreed upon. Once the sizer is filled, the operating table will be moved to a seated position. I do this so I can evaluate your breast's appearance in an upright position. Once your breast looks as perfect as possible, I return the operating table to the flat position and remove the sizer.

Next, I carefully examine the inside of the breast pocket to ensure no bleeding (called hemostasis) has occurred inside the pocket I created. Once I've confirmed hemostasis, my team and I move to the next step.

RE-PREPPING

This means I clean the breasts again with a surgical-grade solution. (See figure 10.2.) I take this additional precautionary step to protect against bacteria or other contaminants that may have reached the skin. I also change and then wash my gloves with an antibiotic solution to kill any microscopic contaminants. Making sure my gloves are sterile as possible is an important step to maintaining the sterility of the implants.

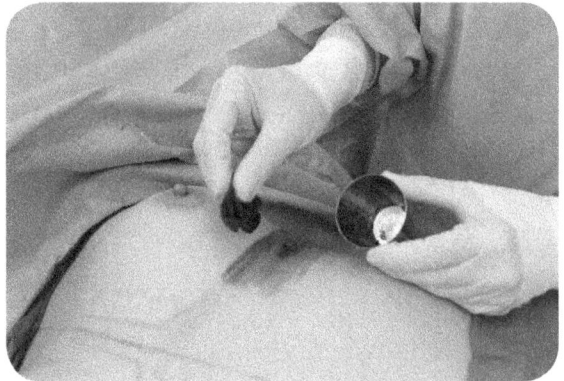

FIGURE 10.2. Re-prepping the skin. Gauze is soaked with a surgical-grade, antibacterial solution, and the skin around the incision is again cleansed.

IMPLANTS: OPENING OF PACKAGE, NO-TOUCH TECHNIQUE, AND INSERTION

Implants arrive at my office in a sterile box. On the outside of the box is an outer seal. My nurse breaks the outer seal, and this allows the box's lid to be opened. Next, the nurse takes out the plastic container holding the implant. (See figures 10.3, 10.4, and 10.5.)

The implant is housed in two additional layers of protection. The nurse must peel away a second seal to reveal the inner container. The inner container has a tab on it. I use this tab to remove the inner

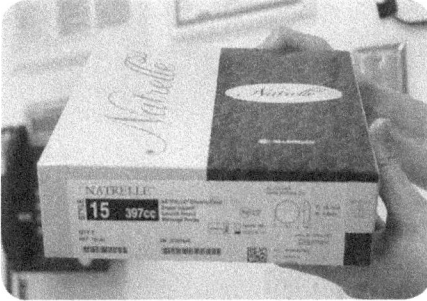

FIGURE 10.3. Implants come in a sealed box.

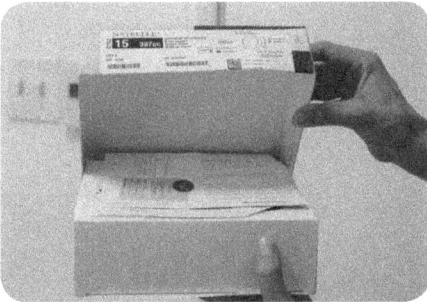

FIGURE 10.4. The first seal on the box is opened by the nurse.

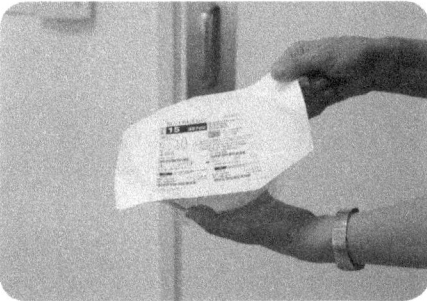

FIGURE 10.5. The container inside is removed by the nurse

container. The implant is kept inside this inner container and is protected by a third seal. I then remove the third and final seal to expose the implant. Now the implant is ready to be used. (See figures 10.6, 10.7, and 10.8.)

In order to maintain the highest degree of sterility of the implant, as mentioned previously, I use a no-touch technique, which ensures the least possible handling and exposure of the implant to the operating room environment. Once the implant leaves the sealed container, I immediately place it in a device called a Keller Funnel,

FIGURE 10.6. I remove the implant from the container using a tab.

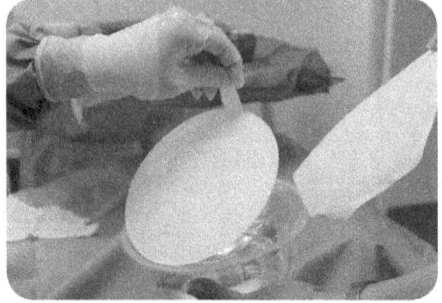

FIGURE 10.7. The implant is inside this inner container.

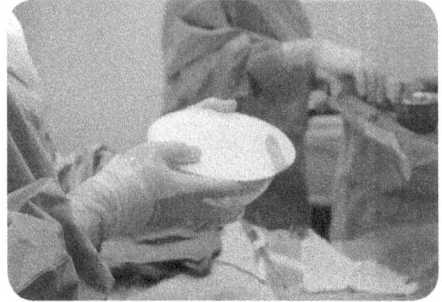

FIGURE 10.8. I open the last seal. The implant is now ready to be used.

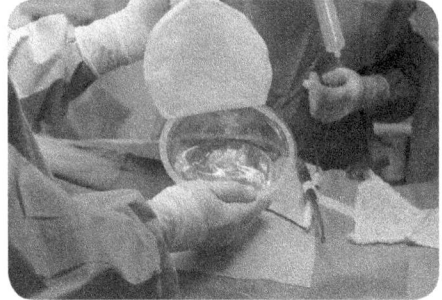

which is an implant sleeve. The no-touch technique combined with the care I take to make sure the implant does not sit uncovered once removed from its packaging minimize micro contamination. (See figures 10.9 and 10.10.)

With the implant inside the Keller Funnel, I use gentle pressure to slide the implant through the funnel, then through the incision, and finally into the breast. (See figures 10.11 and 10.12.) Next, I place the operating table in the upright position once again to evaluate the breast's appearance. I carefully review the breast's shape and size and

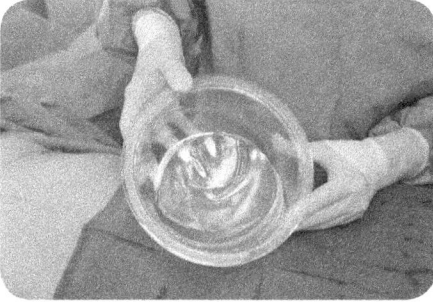

FIGURE 10.9. The implant is located inside the inner container.

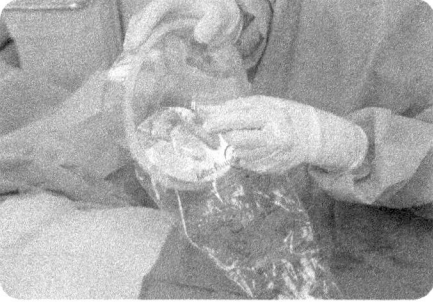

FIGURE 10.10. The implant is then transferred into the implant sleeve.

make minor adjustments if necessary. I again ensure that the breast looks as perfect as possible. After the breast has passed my review, I return the table to the flat position.

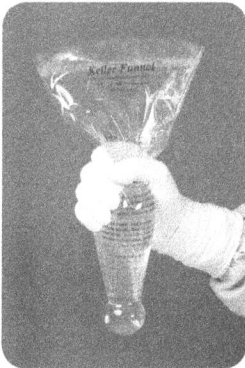

FIGURE 10.11. The implant is now inside the implant sleeve.

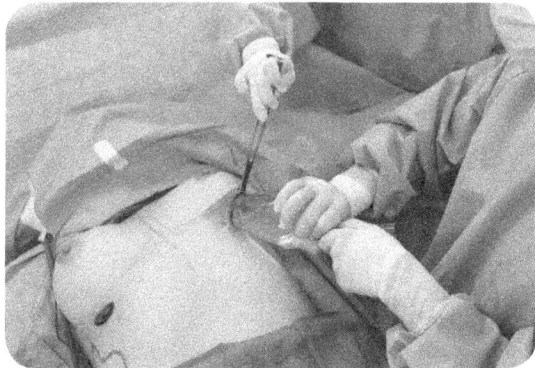

FIGURE 10.12. The implant sleeve is used to gently insert the implant into the breast.

OTHER BREAST

From the local infiltration to implant insertion, I then repeat the entire process for the other breast. After the sizer is inserted in the second breast, I perform an additional examination to ensure both breasts are as symmetrical as possible in size and shape. This step is repeated after the actual implant is inserted as well. These multiple evaluations make sure the breasts look as beautiful as possible.

CLOSURE OF INCISIONS

Once the implants are in place, I then close the incisions. They are sealed using numerous delicate and absorbable stitches, which precisely align the multiple layers of skin (the epidermis, dermis, and fascia) so the scar heals as thinly as possible and only a fine line remains.

Next, I apply a thin layer of adhesive over the incisions. Special small, thin, white cloth tape, called Steri-Strips, are used to cover the incisions. I also apply sterile gauze.

BRA PLACEMENT

Once I've covered all the incisions, I place a soft supportive bra on your breasts. This bra provides gentle support for your breasts during your initial recovery. This step marks that the procedure is now done. The surgery itself requires between forty-five minutes to an hour.

Post-Surgery: Emergence from Anesthesia and the Recovery Room

Now, your anesthesiologist begins to reduce the amount of medications and gases he or she delivers to your body. The anesthesia slowly tapers off, and you begin to wake up.

The anesthesiologists I work with are experts at serving patients who are undergoing breast augmentation. This means they know exactly how much anesthesia to administer and when to begin reducing it in order to make sure you wake up as smoothly and comfortably as possible.

THE RECOVERY ROOM

Once you've emerged from anesthesia, you're then taken to the recovery room (see figure 10.13). In the next chapter, we will cover in more detail what you can expect and how you need to prepare for this transitional time.

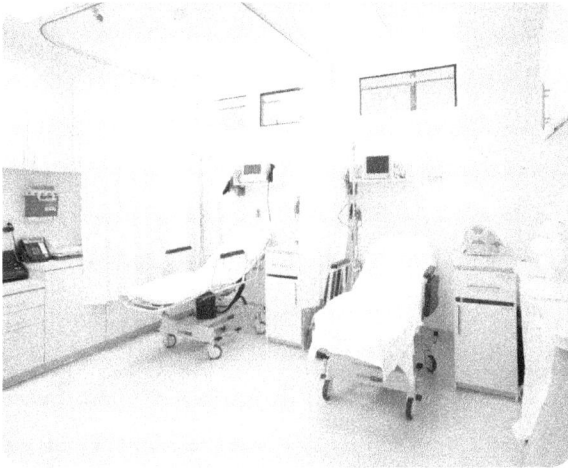

FIGURE 10.13. The recovery room.

Throughout this period, our nurses will monitor you and ensure you're taken care of. If you require extra medications, they will administer them. Once you feel you're ready, my nurses will locate your belongings and help you dress. My team will gently transfer you from the recovery bed to a chair.

My nurse will then review all medications and postoperative instructions with you and the person accompanying you. My goal is to ensure the highest level of patient communication. Thus, my team and I will make sure you understand what you'll experience and what you'll need to do during the next few days.

The person responsible for picking you up and taking you home is now allowed to do so. This family member or friend usually drives his or her car to the enclosed private parking area located directly in front of the elevators to my office. The nurse transports you to the area. Once the nurse has made sure you're safely inside the car and comfortable, you are released to return home.

As you've read, there are many steps to having breast augmentation. I'm proud of my track record of success, which is one reason I have one of the nation's busiest cosmetic surgery practices. In order to meet my high standards consistently, I use the most effective, efficient methods in my breast augmentation approach, which you've read about in this chapter.

Summary

- The total time you will need to spend in the surgery center on the day of your procedure is approximately three hours.

- Usually, patients need to arrive at least one hour before their scheduled surgery start time.

- Breast augmentation takes approximately one hour to complete.

- Anesthesia during breast augmentation is very safe.

- Excellent surgeons use advanced techniques to ensure you have the best results. This includes using a no-touch technique for the implants.

- Patients generally recover in the facility for about an hour before being allowed to go home.

Now that we've explored your surgery, your recovery begins. In the next chapter, you'll receive a day-by-day overview of the recovery process.

Breast Augmentation Myths

> Breast augmentation surgery is only about an hour long, so I should be in and out of the office in around an hour and a half.

Although your surgeon may complete your breast augmentation within one hour, you'll need to schedule about three hours for the entire procedure. The additional time is necessary for steps that must be taken before and after surgery. Every step has been designed to ensure your surgery is safe, is as pleasant as possible, and provides you a beautiful long-term result.

> Breast augmentation surgery is done in a hospital.

Most elective procedures, including cosmetic surgery, are performed in an outpatient surgery center. Outpatient surgery centers are facilities that have all the necessary supplies and equipment of a hospital operating room but are located apart from a hospital. Given the changes in healthcare, the use of a hospital operating room is now prohibitively expensive, especially for elective cosmetic surgery.

Some plastic surgeons, including me, build surgery centers within their offices. In order to build a surgery center, the center must be approved by one of several national organizations in the United States. These organizations carefully scrutinize and inspect outpatient surgery centers to ensure they uphold the highest standards of patient care.

Once approved, the surgery center is given permission to be used as an operating facility. For example, my operating suite is approved by the American Association for Accreditation of Ambulatory Surgery Facilities (AAAASF). This stamp of approval guarantees that my operating room and recovery room have all the equipment, supplies, and medications needed for surgical procedures. It also ensures that my facility follows all the rules and regulations to provide excellent patient care.

CHAPTER 11

THE RECOVERY

In this chapter, you'll learn:

- what you can expect during the recovery process at each stage;

- the steps you must complete the days, weeks, and months after your breast augmentation;

- common postoperative issues most patients experience after surgery.

Real Conversations

When Kimberly was searching for plastic surgeons online, she was drawn to Dr. Wilson's "Flash Recovery Breast Augmentation" that he promoted on his website. As a result, she phoned his office and scheduled an appointment.

During her consultation, the doctor promised a twenty-four-hour recovery period. This appealed to Kimberly because she was a waitress who had very limited time she could take off from work. With Dr. Wilson's procedure, she would be able to undergo her operation on Friday and return to work on Monday.

On surgery day, Kimberly's breast augmentation went smoothly. It was Friday, and she returned home and rested. When she woke up on Saturday morning, she was more exhausted and sore than she had expected. Despite this, she held on to the promise of Dr. Wilson's promoted recovery time.

To Kimberly's dismay, on Sunday she was still sore and tired. With work less than twenty-four hours away, she knew that weaving through the restaurant's dining room serving customers would be impossible.

Although she dreaded phoning her boss to request Monday off, she had no choice. And to make matters worse, during her call she also let her manager know she might not be able to work her next shift or the one that followed. Her boss wasn't pleased, and she knew the unexpected time off put her job at risk.

As each day passed after her surgery, Kimberly became increasingly frustrated with Dr. Wilson's false claim. She phoned her best friend to express her discontent. "I wish he'd been honest with me and told me there'd be no way I'd be fully recovered in twenty-four hours. I feel as if he tricked me so I'd schedule a surgery right away. If I'd known how long it would take, I probably would have waited for a better time to have my surgery," she said.

Introduction

As the saying goes, "if it sounds too good to be true, it probably is." This applies to multiple aspects of our lives, including breast augmentation. Kimberly's experience demonstrates that slick marketing tactics can provide misleading information.

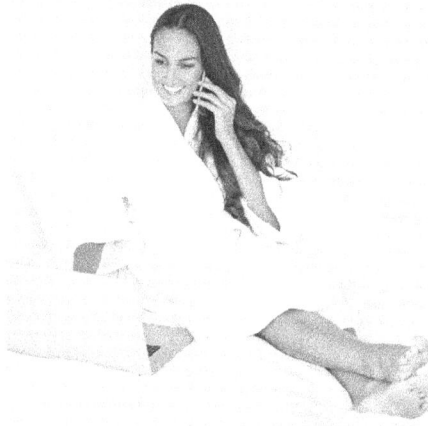

In the end, a twenty-four-hour recovery from breast augmentation does not exist. This is because no matter how skilled the doctor is, he or she cannot change the reality that breast augmentation is surgery that requires a few days of recovery time. Kimberly's example points to the consequences women face when their surgeons over promise and under deliver.

In my case, I regularly work with women who have demanding jobs and jam-packed schedules. And many have young children to take care of. For these patients to arrange time off to undergo and recover from a breast augmentation is no easy task. This is one reason I make it a priority to provide realistic information regarding the recovery period—if I set unrealistic expectations, my busy patients would be highly inconvenienced.

In this chapter, I'll provide you the same detailed information I share with my patients regarding what to expect and how to best prepare for the postoperative recovery period. You'll also learn what activities you can and cannot participate in during the days that follow your surgery. In the end, the more you know and prepare, the smoother your recovery will progress.

As you read the following sections, keep in mind that I'm

describing the process most women will go through. This means some patients will recover faster and others will recover slower. With that said, the sections "Immediately after Surgery" and "First Day after Surgery" reflect experiences nearly all women have. Also, similar to what I presented in the previous chapter, the information you'll read here is specific to the surgeries I perform.

In other words, while all doctors are trained to provide safe medical procedures and all top plastic surgeons share similar strategies, every physician has a particular way in which he or she performs a breast augmentation. Thus, it would be impossible to account for every surgeon's approach. At the same time, the stages of recovery you'll read about are common to women who undergo a breast augmentation with any highly qualified plastic surgeon.

Immediately after Surgery

Once you leave the operating room, you'll spend about an hour in the recovery area. Typically, you'll require about forty-five minutes for most of the anesthesia to wear off. As it does, you'll begin to feel more awake, more alert, and stronger. If a family member or friend is waiting for you, he or she is allowed to visit you in the recovery room at this point.

Due to the pain-relieving medications you were administered, you'll most likely experience only mild discomfort the first couple of hours after surgery. But you will feel significant drowsiness and fatigue, which makes driving unsafe. This is why you need to have someone you trust pick you up from my office.

Some patients experience nausea after surgery. This is one of the side effects of the medications. Rarely do my patients reach a point where they vomit, but this is always a possibility. In order to decrease nausea, you should move as little as possible after your procedure.

While most of my patients live within driving distance of my

Beverly Hills office, some patients arrive from other states and countries. If you live outside the Los Angeles area, I highly recommend you stay in a hotel near my office for the first twenty-four hours after surgery. That way, your car ride from my clinic to your hotel room will be as short and convenient as possible.

Once you arrive at your home or hotel, your number one priority is rest. Lying in bed or relaxing on a comfortable couch is best. You should not lift or push anything heavy. You'll most likely feel well enough to prepare a simple meal, move around the house a bit, and use the bathroom.

At this point, you'll begin feeling physical discomfort. This is why having the pain and muscle-relaxing medications you picked up prior to the surgery day is so important. Patients often tell me they took their pain pills and muscle relaxants as soon as they began experiencing pain, and doing so kept them comfortable.

Because of the medications in your system and your body's healing process, you'll most likely spend the remainder of the day napping and resting. You'll probably be able to walk around on a limited basis, but you should still rely on a trusted person to stay with you to provide assistance in case you require it.

The night after surgery, you'll probably fall asleep quickly. Some of my patients tell me they woke up repeatedly in order to adjust their bodies because certain sleeping positions caused discomfort. To increase comfort during bedtime, I recommend keeping your head and chest slightly elevated by placing two to three pillows behind your head. This helps reduce swelling and pressure against the breast.

First Day after Surgery

You may feel more pressure and soreness in your chest area on the first day after surgery because the medications you were administered during surgery will have worn off by this point. In addition, the following day your body will experience more swelling, which will cause more pain, pressure, and soreness.

Next, the two sides of our bodies heal differently. Typically, one breast will feel more painful than the other. In addition, one breast will experience more swelling and bruising than the other. These differences will diminish, but you'll need to wait several weeks for this to happen.

You can take the pain medications you were prescribed every four to six hours. On the first day after surgery, you should plan on resting as much as possible. You should still avoid lifting or pushing anything heavy during this time. You'll probably have enough energy to prepare something simple to eat, move around the house, use the bathroom, and do other light activities.

You are free to shower the first day after surgery. But most of my patients decide to wait until the second day because they prefer to spend the entire first day resting. If you choose to shower, be sure to remove the support bra that was placed on you after surgery.

Beneath the support bra are watertight bandages covering your incisions. With these in place, your breasts can safely get wet. But you should avoid soaking in a tub or rubbing soap near or on the incisions. Once you're done showering and have thoroughly dried your breasts, be sure to place the support bra on right away.

Because you'll still feel tired and drowsy, I recommend you spend the day resting and relaxing and you limit your activities to reading or watching movies or TV.

After the first night, you don't need to sleep with the support bra on. But most patients prefer to continue wearing it because they feel more comfortable with the support the bra provides.

Second Day after Surgery

Although some pain, soreness, and pressure will continue, most patients start feeling better after the second day. Pain and muscle-relaxing medications taken at regular intervals will continue to help with recovery and healing.

If they did not shower on day one, most patients will do so on the second day. As mentioned before, remove the support bra to shower and let soap and water fall on the breasts. The incisions will be covered with a watertight tape for protection. You should not rub the incisions, however, or soak in a tub.

The breasts will have some bruising, obvious swelling, and will appear high on the chest. Also, one breast may be more painful and appear more swollen, higher, and more bruised. This difference between the two breasts will be particularly apparent the first few weeks after surgery. Over time, the breasts will appear more symmetric. Although you should remove your support bra to shower, I recommend wearing it as much as possible throughout the day.

The second day, you will still feel a little tired and drowsy. Most patients continue to rest as much as possible. Again, reading in bed and watching TV or movies on the couch will be the best way to spend your day.

In regards to tasks associated with work, such as texts, emails, and phone calls, keep in mind you'll most likely still be on pain medications, which could affect your thinking and judgment.

Third Day after Surgery

This day usually signals a marked decrease in pain and an increase in energy. Muscle relaxants are usually no longer necessary after the third day, and most patients decrease their pain-pill intake.

On the third day, you may feel well enough to leave the house. While driving on your own is premature, being a passenger is fine. Many of my patients have enough energy and strength to eat out, window shop, catch a movie, or participate in another relaxing activity.

If your job allows and it's not physically demanding, you may be ready to work from home by this point. This includes reviewing documents, emailing, and making phone calls. You should still avoid lifting and pushing anything above four or five pounds.

Keep in mind your energy level will still be low. Thus, I advise against returning to the workplace or school, unless you're able to arrive and leave whenever you want.

Regardless of how you fill your day, you should commit to arriving home early to rest. And I also recommend remaining flexible with your plans. In other words, give yourself the ability to return home at any point during the day if you feel tired.

You should plan on making this day as light as possible. Going out and participating in simple activities are okay. But make sure to keep your activity to a minimum. In fact, your overall recovery will be better if you focus on resting the first few days.

Fourth Day after Surgery

On this day, you'll probably still experience discomfort—but less so compared to prior days. Although you may experience pain, your mobility, strength, and flexibility should increase, and your pain medication intake should decrease.

Similar to day three, you'll probably feel well enough to spend time outside the house, perform low-key tasks around the house, and work—as long as it doesn't require heavy lifting or pulling.

Fifth and Sixth Days after Surgery

By now, the vast majority of my patients don't need any pain medications. They're feeling stronger and more mobile with each day that passes. At the same time, certain sudden movements, particularly in the upper body, may cause discomfort.

You should be able to drive at this stage, as long as the medications you're taking aren't impairing your ability to do so. Also, you may feel well enough to return to work or school—as long as no heavy lifting or pulling is involved.

Even if work or school is not physically demanding, you'll probably notice decreased stamina compared to how you felt before you took time off. That's why, if your schedule permits, I recommend avoiding work or school on the fifth and sixth days.

One Week after Surgery

The seven-day point marks your first follow-up appointment with me. In regards to patients who live in other states and countries, I require at least one week be spent near my Beverly Hills office after the breast augmentation. I insist on this so that we can meet for your first follow-up appointment. If, after the follow-up appointment, you're healing well, then you can return home confident your procedure went as planned.

SUMMARY OF RECOVERY

Days 1–7

DAYS 1-2
Rest, can shower, do light activities around the house

DAY 3
Less pain, more strength, more energy; can go out

DAYS 4-5
Return to light work, school, maybe driving

DAY 7
First follow-up appointment

The follow-up meeting serves two important functions:

1. I'll listen to your questions and concerns.

2. I'll examine your surgical results, which includes taking photos to document your progress, and ensure you're healing properly.

During the appointment, patients often express concerns about swelling, tightness, a "high" position of the breasts, and asymmetry.

Swelling should still be expected at this point. The affected area is usually concentrated over the top of the breasts.

In addition, the breast skin may feel tight, and this tautness may slightly push the implants upward making the breasts appear high. Both the tightness and upward appearance will diminish once the skin around the breasts relaxes in order to accommodate the implant.

In regards to asymmetry, previously, you learned each side of the body heals slightly differently. Thus, one breast may appear higher than the other, and one breast may be more swollen, bruised, or hurt than the other.

Swelling, tightness, an upward appearance of the breasts, and asymmetry are all expected outcomes after breast augmentation.

During your exam, I'll perform a thorough evaluation to ensure your body is healing well. I'll remove the special waterproof bandages I placed over the incisions. Below the incision, within the skin, is where the stitches are located. Your body will eventually absorb these. On occasion, I may need to trim some stitches. This is painless. Once I can see your incisions, I make sure the scars I designed meet my standards of excellence.

All scars need time to heal properly. Initially, your scars may appear slightly thick and red. Over the weeks and months that follow, this thickness and discoloration will diminish. Scars usually require six months to a year to fade. You can apply scar creams after the first week to speed up the healing process.

BREAST MASSAGES

I usually recommend patients begin breast massages one to four weeks after surgery. Think of the following four types of massages as physical therapy designed to improve the outcome of your breast augmentation. I advise carrying out the four exercises in succession at least three times a day. You can perform them more often if you're able. Completing them consistently over several weeks will help reduce swelling and pain, and your breasts will become softer.

Notice this information appears in the "One Week after Surgery" section. This is because I advise waiting at least one week, if not more, before beginning the massages. Prior to a week, your breasts will be too tender and sensitive to properly massage them. In addition, there is no added benefit to performing these massages any sooner.

1.   Place your hands on the outside of both breasts. Next, push your breasts together so they meet in the middle of your chest. Complete ten repetitions of this. Initially, you may not be able to push your breasts together entirely. But as you recover and continue this exercise, the range of motion will increase.

2.   Place your hands beneath your breasts. Then push your breasts upward as much as you can (stop once you feel discomfort). Repeat this ten times.

3.   Place your hands at the top of the breasts. Then, while applying pressure, slide your hands down your breasts. Repeat this ten times.

4. Cover your right and left areolas with your right and left palms. Then use your hands to squeeze the entire breast including the implant inside. Next, while maintaining your grip, move your breasts in a clockwise or counterclockwise circle (the direction doesn't matter).

SUPPORT BRA

You should continue to wear the support bra you were provided with. It is not necessary to wear it at night. But I do recommend you wear a bra for most of the day. Some patients prefer to buy their own support bras after surgery. This is okay as long as the bra is not tight and does not push the breasts and the implant against the chest. Also, the bra must not contain an underwire. An underwire will be uncomfortable and may irritate the incision.

RESUMING DAILY LIFE

Most patients feel well enough to return to work or school after a week. You may also feel energetic enough to resume exercise. If you decide to go to the gym, avoid upper-body and high-impact workouts. In other words, stay away from lifting or pushing weights that work the arms and chest and intense classes. If you're eager to lift weights, focus on leg exercises.

I recommend resuming physical activity gradually. Walk on the treadmill or use the StairMaster or an elliptical machine on a gentle setting. Avoid running or jogging, no matter how low impact you think it is. As your recovery progresses and you begin to feel stronger, you can gradually increase your physical activity.

I discourage sunbathing for another two to three weeks. Sun exposure and tanning beds will increase swelling of the breasts. Also, the ultraviolet rays interfere with scar healing and cause scars to appear darker and more noticeable than would otherwise be the case. Thus, if the breasts are exposed to the sun, patients must apply sunblock to the skin and to the scar. The scar should be covered as well if there is a chance of sun exposure.

Many of my patients travel from other states or other countries to undergo surgery with me. The minimum amount of time that must be spent in the Los Angeles area after surgery is one week. As long as everything appears to be healing well, patients are allowed to travel after this first appointment.

Two Weeks after Surgery

By this point, you'll be pleased with the noticeable reduction in swelling and bruising. In fact, all bruising may be completely healed at this stage. The breast skin will have relaxed to where you'll notice the breasts take on a more pleasing shape.

You may still feel chest soreness and discomfort, but these are usually restricted to specific movements or actions. Also, one breast may still hurt more than the other—this will continue to improve in the weeks ahead.

In regards to physical activity, you still should avoid heavy lifting or pushing that uses your upper body. Also, activities you participated in before your breast augmentation may seem harder to do now. This is a normal part of the recovery process.

Participating in activities or jobs that involve lifting or pushing relatively light objects is usually okay by this point. When trying, however, you may still feel slightly weak. I advise against any heavy lifting or pushing. If you must perform heavy lifting—for instance, because you're raising small children or it's part of your job—make sure to have someone nearby who can help if needed.

Overall, if you experience any discomfort during physical activity, listen to your body—it's telling you to slow down and lighten up. Remember, you'll have plenty of time to resume your normal routines.

Three to Four Weeks after Surgery

Most of my patients feel great at the three- to four-week mark. They're excited to see swelling decrease, and their breasts take on the shape they had looked forward to. They've resumed most of their normal routines, including gym workouts, and physical discomfort is mild and limited to only certain movements.

SUMMARY OF RECOVERY

1–4 Weeks after Surgery

WEEK 1
Full return to work, school

WEEK 2
Can increase activity at gym, use light weights

WEEK 3
Increase activity at gym; can use heavier weights
Swelling continues to decrease
Breast skin begins to relax

WEEK 4
Second follow-up appointment

In regards to exercise, light jogging and swimming may be possible at this point. And you may feel strong enough to begin weight lifting that focuses on the arms or chest or both. You may still feel weaker than you did prior to your breast augmentation. This is normal and will improve over the following weeks.

At the three- to four-week mark, many of my patients feel well enough to take short trips. Sunbathing is also fine at this point. Sunblock, however, should be applied to the breasts, especially over the scars. In fact, sun exposure to the scar should be strictly avoided for at least six months.

Your second follow-up appointment usually takes place at this point. The purpose of this visit is to address your questions and concerns and make sure you're healing well.

If I'm satisfied with the outcome of your breast augmentation so far, I'll let you know you're free to stop wearing your support bra, and you can wear any type of bra or clothing you choose. At the end of your appointment, I'll take photos in order to track the progress of your recovery.

Three Months after Surgery

The next follow-up appointment is three months after surgery. The breasts are now usually fully healed and settled. Scars are significantly improved and may be inconspicuous. The breasts usually look their best at approximately three months.

Patients have fully resumed all activities by this point. Any minor issues, such as discomfort or mild asymmetries, have usually resolved by now. The appointment is used to answer any remaining questions and address concerns. Pictures are again taken.

Six Months after Surgery

While the six-month appointment is optional, many patients look forward to it because they are able to review their before and after photos—the beautiful transformation is exciting for both of us to see. During this appointment, I'll also answer questions and concerns.

One Year after Surgery

This is usually the final appointment. The purpose of this meeting is to make sure your breasts, including the scars, have healed properly. I also take this opportunity to review with you your overall experience and answer any remaining questions or concerns you have.

SUMMARY OF RECOVERY

1–12 Months after Surgery

MONTH 1
Full return to all activities
Can wear any type of bra/clothing
No restriction on travel
Very little swelling of breasts
Breast skin more relaxed

MONTH 3
No swelling of breasts
Breast skin fully relaxed
Scars begin to fade

MONTH 6
Scars continue to fade

MONTH 12
Last follow-up appointment

Common Postoperative Issues

So far, you've learned what you can expect at each stage of your recovery. I've addressed common issues that arise in the subsequent days, weeks, and months after your breast augmentation. In this section, I'll highlight the following issues that can occur at any stage during your recovery:

- Asymmetry

- Sloshing sensation

- Weakness

- Implant awareness

- Animation displacement

- Mondor's cord

The reason you can experience these at various stages is a result of the body's healing mechanism.

ASYMMETRY

First, let's explore asymmetry. As you've learned previously, the right and left sides of the body are asymmetric. Although we have two eyes, ears, arms, legs, etcetera, if you looked closely, you'd see differences between the left and right versions of your body parts. This asymmetry extends to our body's healing mechanism as well.

Even though the same surgery was performed on both sides in precisely the same way, the left and right sides of your breasts will heal slightly differently: One breast may hurt less than the other, one may have less bruising, and one may look higher than the other. These differences may cause one breast to appear bigger—this is normal and experienced by nearly every patient.

In regards to overall sensations, one breast may experience feelings that don't occur in the other breast. For example, you may feel a pulling sensation or sudden sharp pain in only one breast. Sometimes pain can switch from one breast to the other. You may also feel numbness in one breast and not the other.

Next, scars may heal differently as well. One scar may heal or fade faster than the other. And one scar may appear darker or thicker.

The good news is that asymmetries in the healing process usually resolve over time. This includes the appearance of the scar. After your recovery is completed, in most instances, asymmetries will be either negligible or gone.

SLOSHING SENSATION

This refers to the feeling or sound that some women notice during the first few weeks after a breast augmentation. A sloshing sensation usually is a result of the implant's movement inside the breast pocket when air or fluid or both are present in it. When the implant moves, it pushes on air or fluid inside the pocket, and this creates a sloshing sensation. This is normal.

During surgery, air and fluid can accumulate inside the breast pocket while the incision is open. This is an unavoidable part of the surgery process. The body typically absorbs the air and fluid over three to four weeks. Once the air and fluids are absorbed within the body, the symptoms will cease.

WEAKNESS

As you've read previously in this book, in most instances, I recommend placing implants below the muscle. In order to perform a submuscular procedure, the muscle must be opened to allow the implant to fit below it.

Initially, the chest muscle will feel slightly weaker. For the first few weeks, you may also have less strength when lifting or pushing objects that require using your upper-body muscles. As they heal, your strength will recover.

IMPLANT AWARENESS

This refers to a feeling that a foreign object is in your breasts. While you may notice this at first, after three to four weeks, many patients

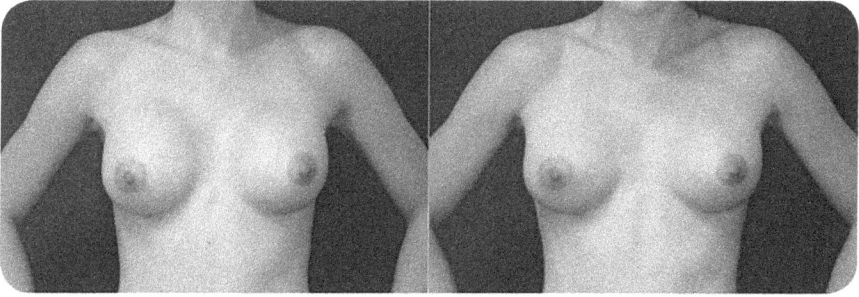

FIGURE 11.1. An example of animation displacement. The picture on the left shows the patient with her muscles relaxed. The breasts have a normal appearance. In the picture on the right, the patient is actively contracting her pectoralis muscles. This causes the muscles to push on the implants and makes the implants move slightly outward.

tell me their breasts feel natural to the point they forget they even have implants.

ANIMATION DISPLACEMENT

Animation refers to the visible movement of the implant within the chest (see figure 11.1). This occurs when the chest muscle is contracted.

When animation displacement takes place, the muscle pushes down on the implant and can cause the implant to move slightly to the sides of the chest. Usually, this is not visible, so only the patient will notice. With that said, animation can be seen with specific movements and when you wear certain clothes. For example, if you lift something heavy while wearing a bikini top, the implant's movement may be visible.

MONDOR'S CORD

This is a harmless and common condition that can occur after breast augmentation. Sometimes after surgery, the veins that run below the breast may scar beneath the skin.

The resulting scar tissue can feel tough and even have a cord-like appearance. In most cases, when the arms are in their downward position, patients aren't aware of this scar tissue. In some cases, however, when their arms are elevated, the scar tissue will be pulled, and it may push up on the skin, and cord-like scar tissue may be visible. (See figure 11.2.) Fortunately, this is harmless. In addition, the scar tissue usually softens over time, and the cord-like appearance goes away without any additional treatment.

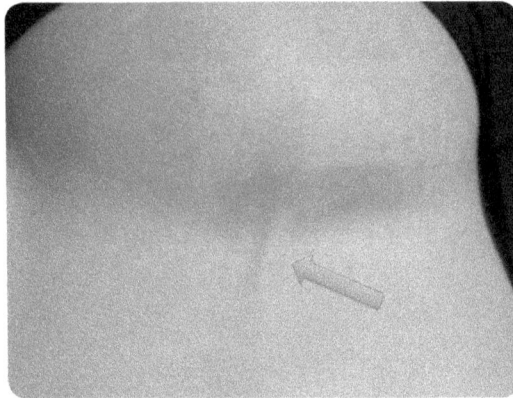

FIGURE 11.2. An example of Mondor's cord. This is a view of the bottom of the patient's left breast while she holds her arms up over her head. In this position, the scar tissue, which is usually not noticeable, can be pulled up. The arrow points to the elevation of the skin in this area. This is harmless and usually goes away with time.

Summary

- Plan on resting for the first two days. Most patients experience some pain, soreness, and pressure for the first twenty-four to forty-eight hours after surgery.

- Symptoms begin to dramatically improve after three days.

- Most patients are able to return to work or school or both after five to seven days. This will depend on how you feel and the amount of physical activity required.

- The first follow-up appointment is usually one week after surgery.

- You can start exercising after one week. But you must start with light activities that avoid heavy lifting and pulling. Gradually increase the intensity over the following three to four weeks.

- Most patients are back to normal after approximately one month.

We've reached the end of our journey. In the final chapter, I'll provide an overview of what you've learned throughout this book.

Breast Augmentation Myths

> I read about a surgeon who specializes in "flash recovery breast augmentations." The doctor says his patients are fully recovered in twenty-four hours.

Throughout my career, I've seen surgeons advertise twenty-four-hour-recovery breast augmentations, and patients have reported hearing about them as well.

No surgeon can provide a twenty-four-hour-recovery for *any* kind of surgery. Unfortunately, this doesn't stop doctors from falsely advertising fast recoveries in order to seize upon women's fears and hopes regarding their breast augmentations.

The human body requires time to properly heal and recover after surgery. While patients can take measures to ensure the process goes as smoothly and as quickly as possible, for surgeons to offer a twenty-four-hour-recovery period is misleading and downright unethical.

Rather than promote a twenty-four-hour-recovery period, I tell my patients they may feel significantly better after twenty-four hours.

When compared to other surgeries, the natural healing process the body must go through is relatively easy after a breast augmentation. Thus, most patients return to their normal daily activities after five to seven days and feel great after three to four weeks.

If a doctor advertises a twenty-four-hour recovery, then buyer beware: The surgeon is showing you he or she is untrustworthy.

In order to plan properly and to ensure an easy recovery, a great experience, and beautiful results, your surgeon must provide honest, realistic information.

As far as my patients are concerned, they frequently tell me their recovery process was much easier and smoother than they had imagined. One reason is because of the thorough preparation they performed prior to surgery day and their strict adherence to my post-surgical guidelines.

CHAPTER 12

THE SUMMARY

Real Conversations

The following is an actual review:

Dr. Diaz is by far the BEST for your surgical needs to look and feel Beautiful & Confident! From the minute I walked in I was greeted with a friendly staff throughout the office! Always very professional and attentive! Dr. Diaz made me feel comfortable and at ease during the consultation, answering any and all questions and concerns I had regarding [breast augmentation]. His knowledge, experience and confidence in being the BEST at what he does truly shows. The technology in his office which helps you to see what your results could look like in your body was a HUGE factor in helping me decide the right size and options for my body. Dr. Diaz gave me his input and suggestions as well which was extremely important. . . . The attention to detail that Dr. Diaz provides is like no other and you have to come see him for yourself to truly understand. Leading up to and the day of my surgery I was constantly put at ease by Dr. Diaz and his staff. I am so happy that I decided to choose Dr. Diaz for my surgery because I Love, Love my results and would recommend him to anyone. . . . Go see Dr. Diaz if you only want the BEST!!

O. D.

Los Angeles, CA

Introduction

Of all cosmetic surgery procedures, breast augmentation is the most common. But this by no means makes it an easy-to-perform surgery. Because the outcome of a breast augmentation will have a significant impact on how you'll look and feel over the long term, you must thoroughly research your options, assess benefits and risks, and learn as much as possible before you undergo it.

In this book, I've provided you an essential guide to breast augmentation. You've learned that when performed by a top surgeon, your surgery can yield a beautiful result that will last for years to come. By reading these pages and following my recommendations, you've dramatically increased the likelihood of experiencing an outcome you'll love. In this chapter, I'll provide an overview of the important points we've covered in our time together.

Pre-consultation

Your breast-augmentation process should begin long before you make an introductory appointment to meet with your prospective plastic surgeon. By the time you phone a particular office, you should have learned the basics about the surgery and asked yourself the essential questions I provided in chapter 1. Review this chapter to determine how to conduct preliminary research.

Research: Finding the Right Surgeon

When it comes to your doctor, the words "board-certified plastic surgeon" are a must-have designation. This means that "board certified" is not enough. While those two words are important, a doctor can be board certified in dermatology, pediatrics, internal medicine, otolaryngology, or any number of other certifications.

Do you want a physician board certified only in dermatology performing your breast augmentation? (The answer should be an emphatic no.) I've witnessed the following unfortunate scenario far too many times: A patient comes to see me for a second opinion because she's not pleased with her breast augmentation outcome. I look the surgeon up online and quickly see he is, in fact, board certified. But not in plastic surgery.

After conducting a couple of minutes of online research, this unhappy patient would have discovered the same information as I did. By doing so, she would have avoided making an appointment to meet with this physician in the first place—let alone entrusting the surgeon with her breast augmentation.

While the power of your smartphones, tablets, and computers means you have countless research tools available to you, these resources can also lead to information overload. In chapter 2, you learned where to focus your time and energy, which will save you time and make your research more efficient. Once you've found surgeons based on the criteria I've provided in chapter 2, I recommend you narrow your list to five doctors. If your area has a limited number of plastic surgeons, you can choose fewer.

Consultation

The introductory consultations you have with your list of plastic surgeons are the best way to learn about your procedure and gather information about each prospective physician. You'll use the outcome of these meetings to identify the best doctor for you. These appointments are an essential part of the breast augmentation process.

In order to make your consultation as effective and efficient as possible, you must prepare for it. Review chapter 3 to identify actions you need to take before you have your face-to-face meeting with your prospective surgeon.

Must-do steps include arriving on time for your appointment, determining what result you seek, understanding the basics of the surgery itself, and knowing how you'll pay for your surgery. When you follow the guidelines I provided in chapter 3, you're doing your part to make the appointment as effective as possible for you.

Implants

You have literally thousands of implant options. If you're like my patients, when you begin exploring your options, you'll feel overwhelmed. Despite the seemingly endless choices before you, in chapter 4, I simplified your search.

You learned that silicone implants and saline implants are equally safe. Despite misinformation about silicone implants, the modern versions of them have a strong outer shell and a thick silicone gel inside to prevent breakage and leakage. They also feel and look more natural than saline implants. For these reasons, most plastic surgeons agree that silicone implants are superior to their saline counterparts.

Implants come in multiple shapes and sizes. Although you have many options, shapes fall into the following four categories:

- Low profile (may also be called "moderate profile")

- Moderate-plus profile

- High profiles (includes high and extra high profiles)

- Shaped-anatomic profile (also called "gummy bear")

Surgeons use these four categories to create a custom result in order to achieve a specific outcome. In general, the moderate-plus and shaped-anatomic profiles provide a natural looking breast, which is what most women seek.

Size

Your implant size is one of the most important breast-augmentation decisions you must make. In chapter 5, I explained in depth how you determine the size that will provide the result you're looking for.

Some patients defer the implant size decision to their surgeons. Others evaluate their size options by using bags of water or rice to mimic an implant. Although both of these are common ways to help you select your implant size, I advise against both for reasons you learned about in chapter 5.

I believe the best approach leverages breakthrough technology. Computer-generated 3D imaging creates realistic and accurate simulations of what your results will look like on your body. This cutting-edge process has made all other methods of evaluating implant sizes obsolete.

Placement

As you learned in chapter 6, you have two implant placement options: above your muscle, which is often referred to as the subglandular position, and below the muscle, which is often referred to as the submuscular position.

While both have advantages and disadvantages, most plastic surgeons agree that the submuscular position creates better long-term results and provides long-term patient safety. Thus the under-the-muscle position is the gold standard.

Incision

Scarring ranks as one of the biggest concerns my patients have when it comes to the final result of their breast augmentation. In order to decrease scarring, several incision options are available to patients.

The four main incisions options are as follows:

- Through the bellybutton

- Through the armpit

- Through the areola

- Through the crease at the bottom of the breast

Each incision point has advantages and disadvantages that I highlighted in chapter 7. I recommend inserting the implant through an incision made at the crease at the bottom of the breast. This incision has been proven to be the best option because it decreases the risk of complications while providing a nearly invisible scar.

Preoperative Process

Once you've selected your implants and have scheduled your breast augmentation, you need to complete the tasks I described in chapter 8. You'll be given informed-consent paperwork to complete, make financial arrangements, arrange time off from work or school in order to recover after your surgery, and have routine blood work performed.

The surgeon's support staff should provide detailed instructions and guidance regarding the preoperative process. You should feel certainty and clarity, rather than doubt and confusion, about the steps you need to take to prepare for your surgery. In fact, your surgeon's office should provide the support and information you need to feel peace of mind throughout the surgical process.

Informed Consent

From root canals to breast augmentations, all surgeries have risks associated with them. The good news is that when performed by a top board-certified plastic surgeon, breast augmentation is a very safe procedure. High-quality surgeons will thoroughly explain risks to you in plain English. In chapter 9, you learned what specific information your doctor should review with you.

The Surgery

All top surgeons know how important this day is for you. They also recognize that reaching this point is both exciting and anxiety inducing for their patients. Your surgeon's processes and procedures are intended to make your surgery as smooth, safe, and relaxing as possible for you.

In the case of my plastic surgery practice, my team and I make sure you're taken care of from the moment you arrive to when you leave. This includes explaining to you, in depth and before surgery day, how you should prepare and what you should expect.

High-quality physicians have perfected every step in the surgical process in order to generate the best possible outcomes. Although I can't speak on behalf of other plastic surgeons, I can attest to how I developed my approach. It's based on creating consistently safe and beautiful results. You learned about my strategy in chapter 10.

Recovery Process

Before their surgeries, my patients often express their concerns about the postoperative process. They're afraid of pain and what their breasts will look like after surgery. But as you learned in chapter 11, in the vast majority of cases, patients later report back to me that the recovery process was easier and far less stressful than they had imagined. This is in large part because we have worked closely together from the start to ensure the surgery meets my standards of excellence.

Most patients spend the first day or two resting and participating in as little physical activity as possible. By the third day, they feel significantly better than they did the first day. My patients often return to work or school and drive their cars after five to seven days.

Results

The following images are of actual patients and their results. (See figures 12.1 through 12.7.)

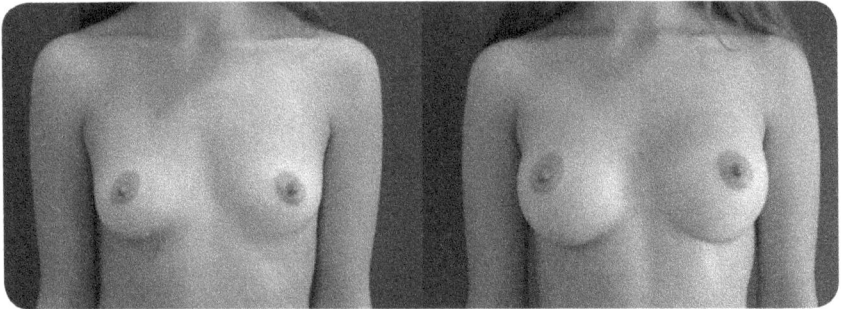

FIGURE 12.1. This patient received silicone implants. The shape is a moderate-plus profile. The volume was 265 cc. The implants were inserted through an incision under the breast. The implants are in a submuscular and dual plane position. Her cup size increased from an A cup to a full B cup.

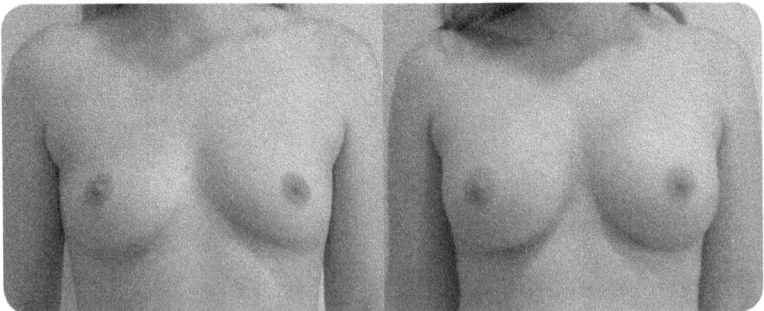

FIGURE 12.2. This patient received silicone implants. The shape is a moderate-plus profile. The volume was 340 cc. The implants were inserted through an incision under the breast. The implants are in a submuscular and dual plane position. Her cup size increased from an A cup to a C cup.

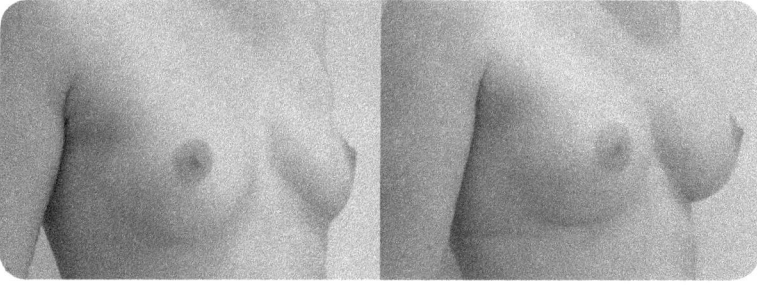

FIGURE 12.3. This is the same patient as in figure 12.2.

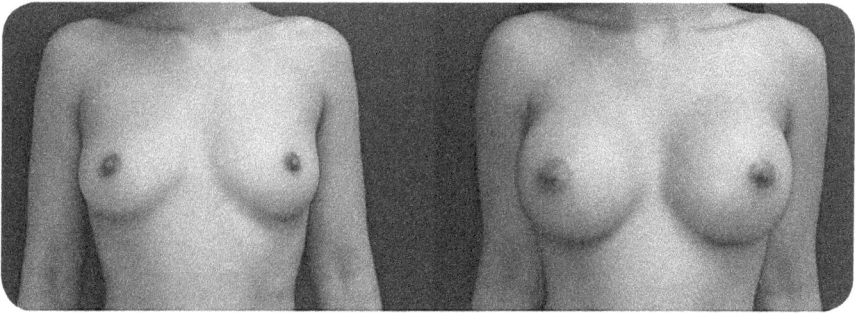

FIGURE 12.4. This patient received silicone implants. The shape is a high profile. The volume was 400 cc. The implants were inserted through an incision under the breast. The implants are in a submuscular and dual plane position. Her cup size increased from an A cup to a D cup.

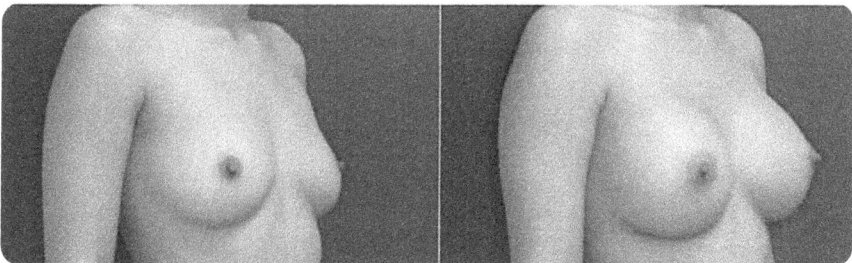

FIGURE 12.5. This is the same patient as in figure 12.4.

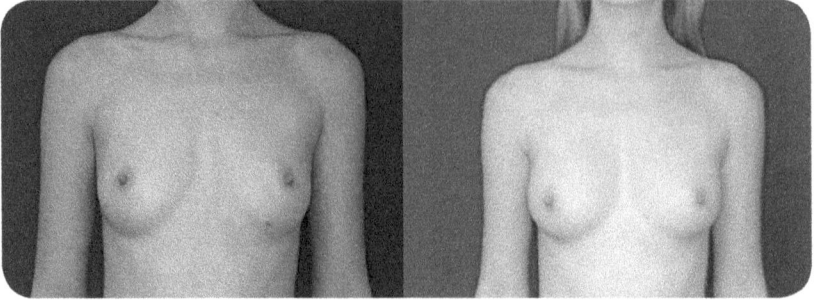

FIGURE 12.6. This patient received silicone implants. The shape is an anatomic-shaped profile ("gummy bear"). The patient had asymmetry in the size of her breasts before surgery. Therefore, different size implants were used to improve her symmetry. The implant in the right breast measured 255 cc. The implant in the left breast measured 185 cc. The implants were inserted through an incision under the breast. The implants are in a submuscular and dual plane position. Her cup size increased from an A cup to a B cup.

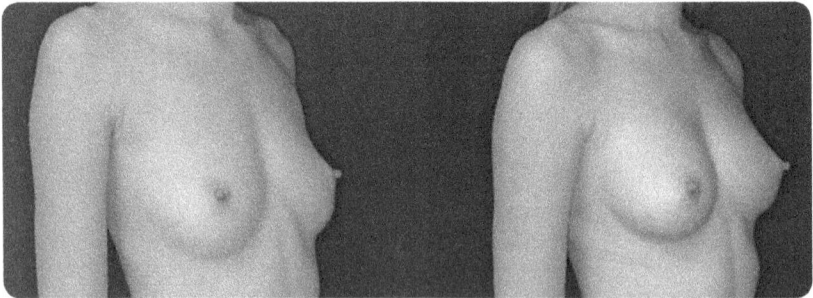

FIGURE 12.7. This is the same patient as in figure 12.6.

Conclusion

At the beginning of this book, I reassured you that by reading these chapters and following my guidance, you'd be a breast augmentation expert. I've taken you through the patient-education process I provide women who come from all over the country and world to meet me in my Beverly Hills office.

Now that you've reached this point, you have the tools necessary to guide you in your search to find the best plastic surgeon for you. Next, I'll tell you what I say to all my patients, "Gather as much information as possible. Educate yourself regarding the different options you have, and seek accurate content."

Last, by following what you've read in this book, you're ready to make the best breast augmentation decisions possible—ones that will provide you the beautiful, long-lasting results you've dreamed of.

ABOUT THE AUTHOR

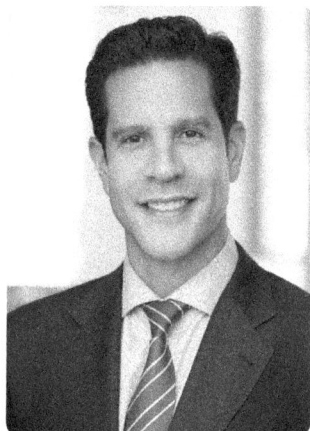

Dr. John Diaz is a graduate of Cornell University and the prestigious Albert Einstein College of Medicine in New York. He graduated medical school with the highest honors, and for this he received the Alpha Omega Alpha Award, which is given to only the top 10 percent of medical students in the country.

While completing his training in plastic and reconstructive surgery in NYC, Dr. Diaz had the privilege of working alongside some of the world's most famous plastic surgeons. His scientific accomplishments earned him a degree with distinction in plastic surgery research.

Dr. Diaz has received awards from the New York Regional Society of Plastic Surgery, Montefiore Medical Center, and the Albert Einstein College of Medicine. In addition to his successful Beverly Hills private practice, he is a medical staff member of the renowned Cedars Sinai Medical Center in Los Angeles, California. He serves as the vice president of the Los Angeles Society of Plastic Surgeons.

As a renowned plastic surgery expert, Dr. Diaz regularly appears on TV and in high-profile print and online publications, such as the

E! network, *Extra, US Weekly,* and *Angeleno.* He has also presented his research results in medical journals and at medical conferences.

By focusing on patient care and consistently providing excellent surgical results, Dr. Diaz's Beverly Hills practice has risen to the top in the nation's most competitive plastic surgery region. In fact, his office consistently ranks as one of the country's highest volume breast augmentation practices.

ORDER BOOKS
AND
LEARN MORE

Now that you've read *A Comprehensive Guide to Breast Augmentation,* visit DrJohnDiaz.com to find additional resources to support you on your journey.

On the website, you can order copies of *A Comprehensive Guide to Breast Augmentation* for friends and family, watch Dr. Diaz's series of YouTube clips about breast augmentation that perfectly complement the chapters in this book, learn about different plastic surgery procedures, and schedule a consultation in his Beverly Hills office.

Dr. Diaz's book is also available at your favorite online booksellers.

You can always get in touch with Dr. Diaz:

> **Web:** DrJohnDiaz.com
> **Twitter:** @DrJohnDiaz
> **Facebook:** @JohnDiazMD
> **Instagram:** DrJohnDiaz
> **YouTube:** DrJohnDiaz
> **Email:** Info@DrJohnDiaz.com

INDEX

A

African Americans, scar variations in, 118
air, sloshing sensation with, 190
alcohol, preoperative avoidance of, 131–132
American Association for Accreditation of Ambulatory Surgery Facilities (AAASF), 172
American Board of Medical Specialties (ABMS), 18, 19, 21, 22, 37
American Board of Plastic Surgery, Inc., 21, 23–24, 36
American Society for Aesthetic Plastic Surgery (ASAPS), 26
American Society of Plastic Surgeons, Inc. (ASPS), 26, 106, 112
anesthesia, 158–159, 158–161
    emergence from, 168–169, 176
    induction of, 160–161
anesthesiologist, meeting with, 158–159
animation displacement, 97–98, 191

antibiotics, 161
anti-nausea medication, 161
anxiety, before surgery, 155–156
appearance of breasts
    desired, determining, 10–11, 75–78
    implant size and, 71–88
    postoperative (results), 187, 202–204
    preoperative measurements and, 44–45
    style (shape) of implant and, 58–67
areola
    implant insertion through, 108, 114–115, 117–118, 121, 145, 200
    width of, 45
armpit, implant insertion through, 108, 113–114, 120–121, 200
arrival
    for consultation, 42–43, 198
    for surgery, 157
Asian women, scar variations in, 118

www.ingramcontent.com/pod-product-compliance
Lightning Source LLC
Chambersburg PA
CBHW030007290326

41934CB00005B/254